Beyond Lectures

Engaging Distance Learning
for Exercise Science and Personal Training

Virginia S. Cowen, PhD

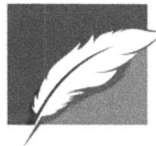

Pennate Press

ISBN 978-1-953891-35-8

Cataloging-in-Publication Data

Cowen, Virginia S., author
Beyond lectures: engaging distance learning for exercise science and personal training / Virginia S. Cowen
ISBN 978-1-953891-35-8
Library of Congress Control Number: 2020923328

Product or corporate names which may be trademarked are included for informational purposes only with no intent to infringe.

First printing December 2020

Published by
Pennate Press
An imprint of IngeniousWellness
P.O. Box 83
Piermont, NY 10968
www.pennatepress.com

Preface

The 2020 coronavirus pandemic had the entire exercise and fitness community scrambling. Personal trainers, fitness instructors, gyms, and studios worked hard to find ways to work with clients. Educators of future exercise and fitness professionals tried to adapt to distance learning by moving lecture content online and saving activity courses for later. Requiring students to be visible on webcam during lectures counted for contact hours. The active aspect of instruction for future exercise and fitness professionals was replaced with sitting and staring at a screen.

One of the most useful things I learned from my years of teaching was that students need to be engaged in learning. Having a sense of belonging was often as important as the contents in a course. In order to foster engagement and belonging, students need to be drawn in. It is hard to do that watching an online lecture.

As social distancing and the need for remote learning dragged on, murmurings started to come from students and instructors seeking something beyond lectures. Instructors had plenty of course material but wanted teaching strategies and help navigating institutional and accreditation requirements around online instruction. Bespoke versions of this book were created for other areas of fitness and wellness. This one, for exercise science and personal training will—I hope—help faculty reimagine and reinvent distance learning offerings.

Virginia S. Cowen, PhD

Contents

CONTENTS

Introduction

Distance learning uses one or more approaches to connect instructor and students in an educational experience that is not in person. Distance learning offers convenience. Students have access to courses and institutions far from home. Time saved commuting to school can be spent on other pursuits. It offers some flexibility. Depending upon instructional format, students can schedule school activities around work and family responsibilities. For many students, distance learning is an appealing alternative to live, in-person instruction.

Distance learning is not always planned. Inclement weather—or a global pandemic—can cause live course meetings to be cancelled. In order to meet requirements for instructional time and contact hours, remote approaches to instruction are needed. Various distance learning formats can be tapped to keep courses and instructional programs on time and on task.

The title of this book acknowledges a trend that took place in the rapid shift to distance learning during the 2020 coronavirus pandemic. Given very little warning, schools and programs had to pivot. Many instructors moved their courses online by delivering live lectures using teleconferencing platforms. A two- or three-hour classroom lecture became a two- or three-hour live online lecture. Requirements that students were visible on webcam counted as contact hours and kept instructors from feeling lonely. Live online lectures provided a low cost way to meet attendance requirements. This remedy kept school in session. But this method of teaching involves more explanation than interaction. The format makes it very difficult to get in-the-moment feedback from students. A live online lecture to a gallery of students viewed on webcams is far less interactive than a lecture held in person.

A phenomenon emerged that became known as Zoom Fatigue (named after a popular technology platform) as instructors and students grew tired of sitting at a computer looking at a gallery of faces on webcams while they listened. Because webcams allow up close views of students, behaviors, postures, and facial expressions that would go unnoticed in a lecture hall became magnified in a virtual classroom. That can be frustrating for instructors who are trying to read a room. At home competition amongst families and roommates contributed to scheduling conflicts to attend remote classes. Prerecorded lectures were offered by some institutions as alternatives to live lectures. This offered flexibility but not opportunity for engagement between students and instructors. The overarching goal for everyone was to keep instruction going even though the format blunted opportunities for connection. Attendance without participation was frustrating for everyone. Fears were voiced about long-term effects of distance learning on student learning outcomes and future professional practice. No one will know how effective it was until students attempt a certification exam—benchmarks for educational programs.

The coronavirus pandemic disrupted education in a positive way by forcing programs to consider what is possible in distance learning. Licensing and certification boards took notice and some relaxed prohibitions against distance learning. As instructors experimented with teaching using webcams, microphones, recorded presentations, and discussion boards, innovation started to emerge. Instead of relying on lectures, or prerecorded content, programs began to seek ways to teach and learn in more interactive ways for engagement. That is possible with active learning.

Across disciplines, it became clear that instructional approaches that were adequate for face-to-face classes were not equally effective online. Even though live lectures and tests met contact hour requirements, they did not make learning stick. Instructional strategies required revision in order to engage students. This book aims to help instructors to re-envision distance learning as something more vibrant and interactive than a gallery of webcams.

This book begins with an overview of post-secondary education to provide context. Regardless of where an exercise science, kinesiology, fitness instructor, or personal training program is housed, administrative practices and accreditation requirements that exist in post-secondary education have a substantial influence on teaching and learning. Understanding administrative policies and procedures becomes critical when major alterations and modifications are made to courses.

Overviews of distance learning tools are provided so readers can see there are many options beyond lecturing. Education technology is part of this book, but technology is not the book's focus. While some companies and technologies are mentioned, the intent is to provide examples and not make recommendations or endorsements. The arena of education technology is rapidly evolving. It would be easy to get lost in a list of websites, apps, and software that could be used to accomplish a task. In many programs and at institutions, decisions on technology are not entirely up to the course instructor so instructors need to adapt their teaching to technology that is available to them. In many cases, there are low-tech possibilities for interactive teaching that can work just as well as a product that must be purchased or requires a subscription. While choices of apps and software is nice to have it is not always required for engaging distance learning. Ultimately everyone needs to work with what they have to design quality educational experiences.

Chapters on course materials, planning, and course structure contain essential information for workload and time management. Balancing class time is important to avoid overloading/under-loading students with work. Instructors must be mindful when changing from contact-hours activity to task-based work. While some of this information is not necessarily specific to distance learning, it is necessary for instructors to consider in instructional design.

Most of the chapters in this book were designed to be short to help instructors find information. The exception is the chapter on Instructional Strategies that forms the meat of the book. Different strategies are introduced and examples are provided to show how instructors can replace live lectures with engaging distance learning activities. For instructors that are not highly familiar with active learning, the detailed lesson plans provided as examples aim to help visualize how a session could be organized in a non-lecture format, for optimal engagement, and meet learning outcomes.

Assessment and feedback is perhaps the most interesting thing that can be different in distance learning compared to a face-to-face class. Distance learning technology offers a wide variety of methods for assessment. Using a range of formal and informal assessments in a course provides opportunities for engagement with—and feedback from—students. Using a broader assessment approach can also provide a more well-rounded picture of overall learning. The book concludes with considerations for implementation for instructors who want to try to move beyond lecturing online to more engaging teaching.

There are a plethora of acronyms used in education. It can be confusing when acronyms are similar, as in team-based learning (TBL) and problem-based learning (PBL.) These sound the same but are different instructional strategies. It can be even more confusing when the acronym is the same for different topics: problem-based learning and project-based learning are both PBL. To help readers from getting lost in an alphabet soup of acronyms, full names are primarily used throughout this book—and acronyms are used sparingly.

Instructors who pick up this book likely recognize that an explanatory lecture is not the only way to teach, nor is it necessarily the best way for students to learn. Those who are willing to reimagine their courses will find practical information to get started. Class sessions that are engaging and interactive can transform distance learning by bringing people back together.

Instructional Formats

Instructional formats can be described in terms of place, space, and time used for teaching and learning. The **place** is where the learners and instructors interact. The **space** includes the way participants communicate with each other and the methods through which the materials are exchanged. This applies to physical space or the tools used to create a learning location in a virtual environment. **Time** provides boundaries for class meetings. Time can include defined days, specific start and end times, or deadlines for when work must be submitted. Often, higher education is thought of as a campus with buildings and designated times for interaction. But it is actually a bit broader because it includes any and all opportunities for formal and informal interaction. Understanding formats for teaching and learning is essential to create optimal environments for distance learning.

Face-to-Face Classrooms

A conventional in-person course is face-to-face learning. This has an established meeting place and specific meeting time for students and instructor(s) to participate in course activities at the same time. Casual interactions can occur before and after class as well as in common spaces on campus allowing for informal exchange of ideas.

Benefits for face-to-face classes are ability to monitor attendance, gauge student attention, and opportunities for students to ask questions and get immediate feedback. It can be easy to pick up cues to identify students who may lack motivation to fully participate in the course or be distracted. The unspoken aspects of communication factor into the experience of face-to-face classes.

Challenges for face-to-face courses include schedule conflicts (for students and instructors) and competition for classroom space. If classrooms are not media equipped it can limit teaching innovations. In classrooms where desks are not moveable, configuring the space for small group work is difficult. During inclement weather, students and instructors may have problems getting to class on time, or at all.

There may be a distance component to face-to-face courses when online technology is used to supply materials and post grades. Students may communicate with faculty via email, but instruction in a face-to-face class does not take place using technology. The boundaries of a face-to-face classroom are more clearly defined than the boundaries of a virtual classroom.

Distance Learning

Distance learning, also called remote learning or online learning, takes place in a virtual classroom. The fundamental concept of distance learning is that instructors and students are not in the same physical location. The virtual classroom provides the place for instructors and students to interact. Virtual classrooms can be configured differently using various technologies that contribute to variety in the space and time for teaching and learning

Distance Synchronous

A **distance synchronous** course does not have an established physical meeting place, but does have a specific meeting time for students and instructor to participate in the course at the same time. Distance synchronous courses can be held using telephone conferences, video conferencing platforms (e.g. Go To Meeting, Zoom, BlueJeans, WebEx, etc.) or live social media (Instagram, Facebook.) Learning management systems have—or can integrate with—live meeting applications. When class takes place in real time, students and instructor are dedicated to learning for a defined period. This can easily count attendance towards contact hours required for a course. In a live course instructors can get immediate feedback on topics or concepts that are unclear. But immediate feedback to instructors only happens when students have the opportunity to ask questions—and get answers—in real time.

Benefits for distance synchronous classes are the ability to accommodate students and instructor from different locations. Time is saved because no one needs to travel to campus. Students who may be reluctant to speak up in a face-to-face class can sometimes be more comfortable asking a question or offering an answer in a virtual environment. Recordings of live course sessions can be saved for students to review.

Challenges for distance synchronous courses are time conflicts, access to technology, and—for some students—availability of internet at adequate speeds. Participation can be a problem for unmotivated students. Students may feel self-conscious about being viewed on webcam. For practical reasons videoconferencing limits the number of simultaneous speakers. It may be difficult for students to ask questions or interact with each other.

Distance Asynchronous

A **distance asynchronous** course does not have an established meeting place nor does it have a specific meeting time. Students and instructor participate in course activities at different times through recorded presentations, readings, discussion forums, chats and assignments. Distance asynchronous courses generally use a course management system, but can also include other methods of communication between instructors and students. Distance asynchronous courses can follow a specified schedule by using sections and deadlines (e.g. 8 weeks with 8 learning units or modules) or allow students to complete course activities on their own schedule within a specified timeframe (e.g. students have one year to finish a course.) There is a wide range of possibilities for place, space, and time in asynchronous distance learning.

The primary benefit of distance asynchronous courses is flexibility: students who work, have families or have other responsibilities can find it difficult fit synchronous courses in their schedule. Being able to choose when they learn can accommodate needs of a more diverse student population. A secondary benefit of distance asynchronous courses is the covert curriculum of personal responsibility. Students must develop time management skills, be accountable, and learn to work in a self-directed manner.

Challenges for distance asynchronous courses include boundaries and flow. Establishing boundaries for completion of assignments and participation in course activities is essential to progress in a course, but can be difficult for students to navigate in the initial stages of a course. The boundaries are essential to ensure course activities allow adequate time to accomplish course objectives. The flow of a course involves not only the material presented, but also the interaction between students and instructor—and among students. Ideally, instructors in asynchronous courses can take a structured approach to teaching that gives students a sense of when they can receive a response to questions, grades for assignments, or other communication from instructors or students. Careful attention to boundaries and flow can help create a smooth distance learning experience for all participants.

Self-paced courses are a special category of distance asynchronous learning. Students view or download course materials and work independently without interaction with other students or the course instructor. The format can be structured for grading—or not. Students can take quizzes or complete activities to earn grades or badges (for non-academic courses.) A self-paced course may be open for access over a defined period of time that includes a start and end date. This type of course may be designed to allow students to have access to all course materials at the start or for new materials and activities to be released on a schedule (a.k.a. **drip content**.)

A primary challenge for self-paced learning is that the students must be motivated to schedule time to engage with the course. Without motivation, students can easily fall behind and become disinterested in completing a course. A secondary challenge is the lack of interaction with the instructor or other students. Students can feel lonely when there is no opportunity to ask questions or exchange ideas with others in the class.

A unique category of self-paced distance learning courses are massive open online courses (MOOCs.) These are open enrollment, distance asynchronous courses that present material to the broadest possible audience. The courses are offered to showcase an instructor or institution. They are often free of charge but are not designed for engagement. Some institutions allow participants in a MOOC to earn academic credit through completion of assessments, application to the institution, and a nominal fee.

Blended or Hybrid

The terms blended and hybrid are used for courses that use a combination of in-person and distance learning. One or more established meetings are scheduled face-to-face for students and instructors to interact in person, the remainder of course uses distance learning technology. The face-to-face portion of a hybrid course might take place at the beginning of the course (to orient students), any point in the course as an intensive/residency, or interspersed with distance learning activities (e.g. alternate weeks.) The distance learning portion of a hybrid course can use either a synchronous or asynchronous approach. A synchronous approach would have students and instructors videoconferencing at usual class time. An asynchronous approach might have students working on small group or individualized learning activities in between—or instead of—live meetings.

Benefits for a hybrid approach are the opportunity to balance in-person meetings with the flexibility of the distance learning component. During the face-to-face portion, instructors can monitor attendance, gauge student attention, and students have opportunities for questions and immediate feedback.

There are several challenges associated with hybrid approaches. Time management can be difficult, especially when the course has an irregular meeting schedule. It may be convenient to meet in person every other week, but that can be difficult to remember. Communication pathways can be confusing. Students may need help figuring out where to go for help—and when. Unmotivated students may struggle to keep up with requirements in the self-directed activities of a hybrid course.

Instructional Format Considerations

Selection of the place, space, and time for a course may be predetermined by the institution. In cases where the instructor can choose the instructional format, familiarity with requirements for the format should be taken into account. Instructors should have training in the use of any technology and adequate tech support during a course when/if things go awry.

Prior to enrolling in a course, students should be provided with comprehensive information about the instructional format, technology needed, and attendance/participation requirements. This includes knowing in advance the schedule for live course meetings, regardless of whether they take place online or in person. A robust orientation is essential to help students—and instructors—navigate the learning environment and recognize where to go for support if problems arise. When/if instructors are tasked with revising the instructional format to a new approach, workload must be taken into account to avoid overloading their schedule.

Post-Secondary Education

Any university, college, vocational, or trade school that provides instruction after the high school level is categorized as post-secondary. Degree and certificate programs in post-secondary education provide specialized instruction. Programs that train exercise and fitness professionals occupy an unusual niche in post-secondary education because programs are housed in different settings that are academic or vocational. Depending upon where the program is located students may receive a degree, diploma, certificate, or certification. In the United States (U.S.), there are five categories of institutions that provide education for exercise and fitness professionals: colleges/universities, community colleges, career/technical schools, proprietary schools, and independent training programs. There are differences across these institutions in size, administrative structure, and accreditation that influence resources instructors may have access to for teaching.

Exercise science and kinesiology programs are offered at public and private **colleges and universities** for graduate and/or undergraduate degrees. Colleges and universities are academically accredited. General education courses (e.g. English, mathematics, and humanities) are required as part of the overall program curriculum. In addition to coursework in basic science and movement science, programs may require students to complete courses in health promotion, behavior, psychology, nutrition, and fitness management. Enrollment in degree programs is competitive admission. Academic courses completed may be used as transfer credits to count towards a degree or certificate in another program at the same college or university or another academic institution. Some colleges and universities also offer nonacademic certificate programs in fitness or personal training.

Community colleges are public, academically accredited institutions that offer liberal arts education in addition to vocational programs and workforce development courses. Exercise science and personal training programs may be offered at a community college for a certificate or an associate degree. General education courses (e.g. English, mathematics) are sometimes included in program requirements. In the U.S., enrollment for community colleges is open to anyone with a high school diploma or equivalent. Some programs at community colleges (e.g. nursing) are competitive admission. But the majority of the degree and certificate programs are open enrollment. Courses completed at a community college may be able to be used as transfer credits to count towards a degree or certificate in another program at the same college or at another academic institution (i.e. college or university.)

Career and technical schools are oriented towards job training and workforce development. Also called vocational or trade schools, the majority of schools in this category are private institutions offering certificates, diplomas, or associate degrees. Schools are licensed by the state where they are located to provide vocational training. Some career and technical schools are specialized and offer training only in related areas (e.g. health professions, cosmetology, or construction trades.) Others take a broader approach by offering programs in health professions, culinary arts, cosmetology, information technology, automotive, fire science, and personal training. Curriculum for programs in this setting is focused on practical skills so general education courses are not required. Application to a program is required prior to enrollment but most schools in this category are non-competitive admissions. A high school diploma or equivalent is required for some—but not all—programs. Courses completed at a career or technical school generally are not transferrable to another institution.

Proprietary schools are private, for-profit schools that provide training for students to earn a certificate or diploma. Proprietary schools include stand-alone institutions or multi-campus institutions with the same name and curriculum. Instruction at proprietary schools is specialized and focused on practical skills like personal training, acupuncture, and massage therapy. Proprietary schools may—or may not—be accredited. Some U.S. states require proprietary schools to be licensed as non-degree granting institutions that provide vocational training. The different types of regulation and oversight applicable to this category mean that there is a wide variety in size and resources in these schools for instructors and students.

Personal training and fitness instructor certifications are also offered through **certification programs** that are not part of the higher education system. These types of programs are similar to proprietary programs in that they focus on practical training and workforce development. Often the aim is to prepare individuals who earn certificates to take certification exams. Examples include courses offered to prepare for the National Academy of Sports Medicine (NASM), American Council on Exercise (ACE) or the National Strength and

Conditioning Association (NSCA) Personal Trainer certification exams.

Accreditation

Accreditation is applicable to some categories of exercise science and personal training education. The U.S. Department of Education currently recognizes 62 different accreditation agencies for higher education. Of these, 26 agencies accredit at the institutional level and 36 agencies accredit programs. The various accreditation agencies assess and monitor standards and quality in education. Each accreditation agency has its own standards. The accreditation process begins when a new institution opens or a new program is launched. It continues at regularly scheduled intervals through a process of internal assessment (self-study) and external review. Any major changes to a course or curriculum—including a change in instructional format—are subject to review by the accreditation agency.

Accreditation for colleges, universities, and community colleges is academic through regional accrediting organizations. The U.S. is divided into six accrediting regions. This type of accreditation is institutional, not programmatic. The review and approval applies to all educational programs at each institution regardless of discipline. Several national agencies accredit career and technical schools. The National Commission for Certifying Agencies (NCCA) accredits several national exercise and fitness certifying organizations including ACE, NASM, NSCA, and the American College of Sports Medicine (ACSM.) This type of accreditation is for the certification program not for educational programs that may be needed to qualify individuals to register for the certification exam.

Teaching and Learning Resources

Depending on the size and category of the institution where an exercise science or personal training program is housed different types of resources are made available to support distance learning. Larger institutions, including universities, colleges, community colleges, and some career/technical schools, use online student information systems to manage applications, enrollment, and registration. They may also offer instructors options for digital management of course materials. These institutions have information technology support departments to support faculty and staff hardware and software needs. This offers infrastructure that can make a migration to distance learning or a hybrid instructional format easier to manage since resources are already in place. Many community colleges have a center for teaching excellence with staff and resources to support teaching and learning. Faculty development workshops in adult learning theory, online course management, or innovative instructional strategies help instructors build knowledge and skills. These centers sometimes have instructional design staff to provide support with development of courses and activities for teaching.

Academic institutions and larger career/technical schools generally have instructional support departments. Staff members are non-classroom educators that work to help all students succeed in school regardless of academic preparation. These departments handle student placement, general advisement, requests for accommodations, and resources for English language learners. These departments also offer test taking workshops, tutoring services, or run peer-tutoring programs. For new students, they may also provide introduction to college workshops to provide an overview of resources, review and other information to help students navigate the LMS and student information system. Any or all of this is important to provide general support to students as well as when issues may arise in distance learning.

The extent to which teaching and learning support is provided in proprietary schools and independent training programs will depend upon the size and scope of the institution. The diversity in configurations of exercise science and personal training programs means that there is no one-size-fits-all approach to distance learning instruction and resources to support general teaching and learning. Some instructors are given wide latitude to learn by doing. This can include experimentation with instructional strategies to find approaches that are well suited to the learning environment and revising when needed. Other instructors have access to instructional designers and technical support, plus they can refer students who need help to dedicated departments.

All higher education institutions, regardless of size, have an area of administration that is responsible for institutional assessment. In larger schools this is a department that conducts institutional research and reviews reports from individual programs. In small proprietary schools this may be a few staff members that review enrollment, grade distribution, and post-enrollment employment statistics. Assessment staff members are also tasked with activities for accreditation. Schools in the different categories are monitored by academic, career, or vocational accreditation agencies for general standards and quality of education. Gainful employment statistics are monitored by the U.S. the Department of Education and can impact accreditation for a school or program.

When a program makes changes to curriculum and/or methods of instruction it may require review on a few levels. Curriculum and instruction committees serve an internal assessment function in colleges and schools. Committee members review new program proposals, new course proposals, and major changes to programs or courses. The focus of the review is to ensure the program or course aligns with institutional goals, follows guidelines, and instructional strategies align with course objectives/learning outcomes. Program and/or course content is compared with similar courses offered by the school to explore duplication of material. Part of the review also includes an evaluation of the course activities in relation to course credit to ensure a balanced workload for students.

Another level of review may involve an accreditation agency. This is generally not necessary when a change is made to a single course, because accreditation encompasses the overall curriculum. When changes are made to several courses, that can constitute a major change which may require accreditation review. Communication internally is essential for quality control of a program. Before making changes to instructional approaches, curriculum, and course content, instructors should ensure that they are following all procedures required for assessment.

Adult Learners

Principles and methods of teaching adults (andragogy) differ in several ways from instructional approaches used to teach children (pedagogy.) Adult students arrive in an educational program with a work and life background and ideas about what they want to get out of an instructional program. Knowles' assumptions about adult learners were that they are ready, motivated, bring experience, have a self-concept, and are problem-focused rather than focused on a topic. Adult students can be self-directed, but they need context and rationale to understand why what they are doing in a class will help them meet their goals.

Principles of pedagogy differ from andragogy in that they assume that students lack experience, are dependent on the instructor for information, and do not have a fully formed identity. Students are not given a choice of topics or any rationale behind material or methods. While children can learn to work in a self-directed manner it is often because they are motivated to achieve a grade or afraid of failure. Instructional approaches are a combination of behavioral and cognitive approaches ranging from explanation, repetition, and review to experimentation, problem-solving, collaboration, and reflection. Complicated topics may be broken down into smaller parts. Foundational material may be integrated with advanced concepts to progressively challenge students.

Motivation to learn can be extrinsic or intrinsic. A student (of any age) who desires to receive praise or achieve a high grade is extrinsically motivated. This type of student is focused on the rewards of the grade. The aim is not to fully engage in learning, but to do what needs to be done to reach a goal. Comparatively, a student who seeks to learn about topic, how it is relevant, and how the topic relates to other ideas or a larger context is intrinsically motivated. The aim is to learn for the sake of learning rather than achieve. An intrinsically motivated student is not focused on praise or a particular grade.

The assumption that all adult learners are intrinsically motivated is faulty in the post-secondary education environment. Even though enrolling in an educational program is voluntary, adult learners may be more focused on grades rather than learning. As students, they may be more apt to skim the surface of course material rather than engaging. This can be more problematic in distance learning which requires students to be self-directed much of the time.

There is an inherent difficulty incorporating adult learning theory into exercise science, kinesiology, and other fitness instructor-oriented programs. Programs have required foundational science courses on topics that students would rather not take. Students might struggle with the lack of choice if they have little interest a topic or have difficulty recognizing relevance. A program might have stringent requirements for contact hours and attendance. If students do not understand or respect the rationale, that can interfere with participation and motivation. All students may not be self-directed, interested in changing social roles, or problem-centered. So the principles of andragogy are not entirely applicable. Adult learners who require context and rationale can have difficulty being motivated and engaged in the full educational program.

A strategic approach for distance learning in any training for exercise and fitness professionals is to draw upon theories and principles from both andragogy and pedagogy. Instructional design that combines explanation and repetition with active learning strategies (problem solving and collaboration) offers opportunities for self-directed learning and engagement. This can be especially helpful for foundational courses to engage students with course material. Review and reflection can be used to help students apply information and understand rationale for material. Frequent assessments that emphasize progress in learning rather than rewards can guide students to becoming intrinsically motivated and engaged in learning as a process.

Distance Learning Tools

Distance learning is instruction that takes place using any method that connects instructors and students in a non-face-to-face environment. Historically distance learning took place in the form of a correspondence course. Students were provided with hard copies of materials. They worked independently to complete readings, assignments, and tests that were returned via mail for grading. Correspondence courses still exist, but the advent of learning management systems brought changes to the space for teaching and learning by providing an opportunity for interaction.

The term online learning is often used interchangeably with distance learning. But there are subtle differences. Online learning refers to a course that is delivered using the internet. Distance learning recognizes that there are different ways to connect students and instructors. Distance learning recognizes the full range of tools that can be used to curate meaningful learning experiences.

Learning Management System

A learning management system (LMS) is an application or platform designed for the management and distribution of online courses. It provides a comprehensive system to handle the complete learning process from delivering content to tracking benchmarks and collecting data that can be used to assess student progress. Some LMSs can be configured to integrate with enrollment management systems to register students and chart progress in a degree or certificate program.

There are a multitude of different LMS platforms on the market as of this writing. Some of the more established companies in higher education include Blackboard and Canvas. Sakai and Moodle are free, open source LMSs that must be customized for use. Other well-known platforms include Schoology, Bright Space, Absorb, and Microsoft's LMS 365, Google Classroom, Securly, Thinkific, Teachable, and LearnWorlds, to name a few. Some of these can be configured as membership groups in addition to offering online courses.

Udemy, Coursera, Lynda, and EdX cornered a unique area of the online instruction market by partnering with higher education faculty and institutions to offer massive open online courses (MOOCs.) Students anywhere in the world can enroll free to participate. Many of these courses offer an option to pay a fee for an enhanced learning experience to obtain a certificate of completion.

A course or content management system (CMS) is more of a repository to support instruction. It contains tools and features manage materials and track student performance. It is generally described as a virtual substitute for a copy machine and handwritten gradebook. A CMS can be used very simply to share materials which support face-to-face instruction. This minimizes the need for instructors to carry piles of student assignments from class to office and back to class after grading. Outside of education, businesses and associations use CMS programs for training and professional development.

The terms LMS and CMS are often used interchangeably. But LMS is generally considered to be more comprehensive for use in an educational program. For ease of reading, LMS will be used in this book.

There are some standard features found in most LMS platforms: calendar, discussion forums, course chat, configurations for units or modules, course roster, and gradebook. The dashboard for instructors and administrators allows control for release of content and tracking when participants log into the course. For instructors, becoming familiar with different tools and features of the LMS can help course preparation and inspiration for creative teaching.

Shareable Content Object Reference Model (SCORM) is a set of technical specifications for development and use of digital learning content. Contents (documents, presentations, videos) can be imported into the LMS or created using features within the LMS. Content that is SCORM compliant can be moved from one LMS to another if an institution switches to a different LMS. Instructors should discuss technical specifications and requirements with instructional design departments or consultants.

Integrations

Digital learning items can be integrated into the LMS or accessed via a link from the LMS. Library or publisher integrations provide access to copyrighted materials in accordance with Fair Use guidelines.

Publisher Digital Assets

Many education publishers have digital resources to augment textbooks. Videos, study aids, integrated media can be accessed by students for assignments or review. Interactive learning environments can replace textbooks or offer students self-paced study and review options. Generally access to digital resources requires rental or purchase of a textbook or a subscription. Educational sales representatives and institutional librarians can help instructors find textbooks with integrated material to use in courses.

Library Resources

Instructors can work with librarians to create resources for courses and programs. High demand items can be placed on course reserves to ensure students can have access. This includes supplemental material, auxiliary content, and journal articles. Subject matter guides can be created to help students find databases and materials for research and writing assignments.

Programs and Apps

The arena of education technology is currently growing at a rapid rate. There are thousands of programs, computer apps, and mobile apps on the market for education. Finding and selecting what to use will be based on functions/features, technological compatibility, as well as where and how it will be used. At larger institutions, instructors may not have any input into integrations. At smaller institutions or independent programs, instructors may be able to make requests for integrated programs or apps.

Popular options include polling software that can be used for surveys or quizzes (Socrative, Poll Everywhere, Turning Point, Kahoot.) Collaboration tools (MindMap, Padlet, Educreations, Doceri) can be used for interactive group assignments. Video production (Snagit, FlipGrid, Inshot) can be used to supply electronic answers to discussion questions or to submit creative assignments. If the program or app will be used during a live online class, students and instructors should be able to toggle back and forth to the virtual classroom.

For active learning, a software program or app should be integrated into the LMS and accessible to all students via computer, tablet, and/or smartphone. Windows, iOS, and android are more popular operating systems, but there are still users of Palm, Blackberry, and others. Every software program or app is not necessarily compatible with all operating systems. Students should be informed of all technology requirements prior to the start of class.

To minimize risk of cheating on tests or quizzes, apps can be integrated that block students from browsing the internet or using other computer-based resources. Once students open a test or quiz, their browser or window is locked and they are unable to open any other apps, software programs, or windows until they finish the test or quiz. Some apps also monitor students via webcam during the test or quiz. A downside of these apps is that they do not work on all devices or internet browsers. Webcam monitoring can run afoul of privacy settings on laptops. If instructors plan to integrate blocking apps during assessments students should be given the opportunity for a test run to work out possible problems in advance of the quiz or test.

Remote proctoring solutions must be purchased for live or recorded audio and video monitoring during tests or quizzes. Blocking apps also require purchase. A low-tech option is to have students take tests or quizzes during a live class session with webcam on so instructors can monitor student behavior..

Gradebook

The digital gradebook in the LMS helps instructors and students monitor progress in a course. The gradebook can be set up with categories of activities (test, quiz, assignment, presentation). A grade and feedback can be provided for each activity within a category. Weightings can be assigned to automatically calculate the contribution of a graded activity or category to the overall course grade. The gradebook can include an option for instructors to return an annotated assignment or qualitative feedback to students in addition to the grade.

A digital gradebook provides an easy way for instructors to validate grades for an activity by reviewing the range, median, mean, and mode for grades. The benefit for students to regularly access the gradebook is the ability to track progress and identify if/when tutoring or additional effort is needed. This is especially important in academic programs for students who excel in lab sessions and demonstrations, but struggle in didactic courses. Students (and instructors) can also see if different types of activities are more challenging than others. That can be useful to help students structure study time and recognize when they might need to seek instructional support. A gradebook is as much a vehicle for communication between instructors and students as it is an accounting tool.

Course Communication

Nearly every instructor has experienced that moment in a classroom when a question asked of the entire class was met with silence. Eyes cast downward; students visibly shrink in their seats. Whether or not students know the answer to a question or have an idea to share, they are reluctant to speak up. Many instructors have encountered the line that forms at the end of class of students who have questions, or perhaps had email exchanges with students who sought clarifications or wanted individualized help. Students may be embarrassed to ask a question in class or they might seek a personal connection. Distance learning can have the same types of problems. This can be compounded by the need for administrative announcements or student advisement. Reminders to students about registration, drop/add, and other administrative deadlines take valuable class time. It can be confusing to sort out where and when communication can best take place.

Recognizing the many pathways for communication is essential to help distance learning run smoothly. Very often a course will use a combination of tools and materials to communicate within the class. This should be distinct from communication between students and administration for non-instructional purposes. When conversations between students and instructors occur in the appropriate place it helps facilitate smooth communication in the course. Orientation to a course should include a section on communication etiquette to inform students on the different communication tool options and how to effectively use them for instructional or administrative purposes.

All course communication that is related to teaching and learning should take place within the course using features of the LMS or via video conferencing. This helps record and archive instructional conversations and also helps students recognize the boundaries of a virtual classroom. Communication that is part of course activity takes place between instructor and students as well as between individual students and within groups of students. Keeping it all in the virtual classroom is the same as keeping the conversation inside a physical classroom—everyone is present and has an equal opportunity to listen or participate.

Communication between students and instructors outside of the virtual classroom should be done for advisement—not instructional purposes. Telephone, email, or video conference conversations are not archived as part of a course. Assistance with a research topic, review of a test or quiz, or general questions about course performance are individualized needs that should take place in private conversations between students and instructors. If communications contain instructional information that is of value to other students it will need to be repeated in the virtual classroom to be fair to all students. Students who seek private instruction via telephone, email, or video conference should be requested to post questions in the virtual classroom or ask questions in class. This insures that the same information is accessible to others in the class.

Forums

A forum is a tool for asynchronous communication using posted information and responses. Effective use of forums requires organization. Students and instructors should be subscribed to all appropriate forums to issue notifications when a forum contains a new post or response. That will help to ensure that all course participants listen to each other. Forums can be used in a course in a few different ways.

General **course announcements** can be posted in a non-interactive forum. This includes information like deadlines for assignments or reminders that are not part of the current course unit or module. A general announcement forum can be pinned to the top of the course page in the LMS so it can be easily found.

Discussion forums can be used for introductions to help students learn about each other at the beginning of a course. Each student can share a short bio or all students can respond to prompt questions. For courses that will be run entirely via distance learning, students could share video introductions, give a tour of their learning space, or demonstrate a unique skill or hobby. If an instructor intends to incorporate video submissions in any assignment, this would give students a chance to experiment with the technology. As the course progresses students can refer back to the introductions forum for information to help them develop an impression of their classmates.

Interactive **discussion forums** are used for conversations and teaching activities. Within a course unit or module, an instructor can start a discussion forum with a prompt, question, or summary of a short assignment. Depending upon how the forum is set up, students can respond with a written answer, video, document, slide set, or something more creative.

The aim of the discussion forum is not to have each student respond just to the instructor, but for all participants to have a robust discussion. The initial prompt should be thought provoking to encourage students to converse with or respond to each other. Discussion forums can be configured for small group or team-based work. Instructors and administrators can view these forums, but students in other groups cannot. These forums basically provide a private workspace within the course.

Course Chat

Students can talk individually with each other or with instructors using chat features in the LMS and/or in video conferencing platforms. In some technologies these conversations can be preserved, but the typical use of chat is for brief exchanges of in-the-moment ideas. In face-to-face courses, chatting is discouraged because the noise and lack of focus can be disruptive. In distance learning, side conversations can take place in a way that does not interfere with class activities.

Phone and Email

Administrative communication is necessary to manage admissions, registration/enrollment, tuition, counseling, career services, etc. So administrative conversations should not take place within course discussion forums or course chats. Separating out administrative conversations from the course naturally occurs when administrators are not inside the same virtual classroom as course activities. But in small schools or programs the instructor might handle all administrative tasks. It can be confusing for students to initiate an administrative conversation in the right place. This also helps avoid losing track of conversations when they are not archived in the right place.

Recognizing that there are different ways for students to communicate with instructors, administration, and other students is essential to keep conversations organized. Instructors may need to repeatedly redirect students to the appropriate communication pathway. This is especially important when a student asks a question or seeks clarification about course content via phone or email. In addition to placing a burden on instructors outside of class time, it is not equitable because others in the class are not included in the conversation.

Collaboration

Collaborative work in distance learning helps foster connections and gives students a sense of belonging. Collaboration helps students develop skills in communication and negotiation. Collaborative assignments give students an opportunity to learn from each other. Because distance learning lacks the opportunity for casual interaction that naturally occurs in face-to-face learning, collaborative work is important to fill a gap. Even though collaborative activities and assignments take time for instructors to create and set up, they place less of a burden on an instructor's time when executed.

Collaboration tools that are used within the LMS or in video conferencing platforms allow students to interact with each other for contributions, mutual accountability, and peer feedback. These tools in an LMS are generally considered to have adequate privacy protections for students. If collaboration tools are not provided, students may seek out other apps or tools outside of the LMS.

When other apps or tools outside the LMS are used, care should be taken to ensure privacy and confidentiality for students and any work they produce.

Selection of collaboration tool for **groups or teams** will depend upon the specific task. Schools that use Microsoft 365 for Education or Google Education have the ability to create collaborative documents, spreadsheets, and presentations. The LMS can be customized to provide discussion groups and collaborative workspace for teams of students working on a specific assignment. A wiki can be used to brainstorm terms, resources and ideas for group assignments—or for the whole class to collect resource material. Some video conferencing platforms (e.g. Zoom, Blackboard Collaborate) have the ability to create breakout rooms for small group work during live sessions.

Simulation is a specific type of collaboration involving role-play or modeling. Participants in a simulation are placed in a real or fictional environment and given a scenario, problem, challenge, or task. Virtual simulation can be done live using webcams for role play. Virtual simulation can also be done online using platforms like VirBELA, Mursion, zSpace, or Open Simulator. Participants create avatars to interact in a virtual environment. Peer teaching is a form of simulation that is often used for active learning. Remote fitness programming during the 2020 pandemic contributed to a great deal of innovation and acceptance of tele-exercise instruction. Programs may want to consider incorporating live online peer teaching into course activities to help students develop skills.

Course Materials

Course materials are any and all contents used for teaching and learning. This includes material developed by faculty, resources on library reserve, electronic textbooks, and integrated media. Distance learning can utilize a combination of digital and hard copy resources. Course materials should take course goal and objectives into account and be selected to support student learning.

Syllabus and Course Outline

The syllabus is essentially a contract for the course that provides an overview and specifications. For distance learning, students can have difficulty getting—and staying—organized. Posting the syllabus and course outline in a prominent place in the LMS is essential.

Providing the syllabus and course outline in advance of the start of a course can be very helpful in distance learning. This allows students to become familiar with the roadmap. They can gain an impression of the overall style of the course and requirements. They can outline the schedule including dates for quizzes/exams and due dates for assignments. Some institutions and programs consider course outlines to be proprietary and do not allow students to access the course outline prior to the start of classes. When this is the case, an audio or video presentation of the syllabus and course outline can be useful to orient students.

Institutional requirements for a syllabus vary, but some of the same essential features are used almost universally. A summary, goal, objectives provide an overview of the course. Rationale for the course—and its place in the curriculum—may be included along with requirements for prerequisites, attendance, and participation. The grading scheme and a grade scale are included so students know criteria for assessment and what constitutes a passing grade. Logistical information is listed including format for instruction, assignments (papers, presentations, group work, etc.) and types of assessments that will be used to measure student learning outcomes. Required textbooks and readings along with recommended resource materials are detailed.

While the syllabus can be considered a course contract, the course outline is a roadmap. It lists the learning activities and schedule for the course. It is customary to design a course in an LMS that works from the top of the page to the bottom. If the units or modules are laid out in a consistent way it can help orient students because it makes it easy to see the shape of a course outline. A separate course outline document may be needed for two reasons: 1) it may be required by the institution to provide a record of course activities, or 2) when course units or modules are dripped (i.e. released individually on a schedule) students will not be able to see the shape of the course until the end.

Together the syllabus and course outline detail what students can expect and what instructors aim to present and assess in the course. For distance learning courses, the syllabus and course outline should be easily accessible for students to help them stay apace and on track. Creating an administrative section at the top of the course page in the LMS can help make it easy for students to find it when needed.

When changes are made to the course outline, the new version should be indicated on the document and the students should be notified that a change has been made.

Instructional Materials

Instructional materials are the contents upon which a course is built. They organize and support teaching and learning. Instructional materials convey information, create space for student engagement through exploration, clarifications, or experimentation, and provide opportunities for assessment. Courses that include required reading and writing assignments are generally associated with learning gains that is expected to be achieved with accumulation and application of information. Ideally, an array of instructional material can be compiled to help students engage with course material.

There are three basic categories for instructional materials: required, recommended, and supplemental. **Required resources** provide the core information for a course. Students must access these materials in order to succeed in the course. **Recommended resources** are optional. They provide students with pre-appraised material that can be used to answer questions or enhance learning. **Supplemental resources** or **auxiliary content** refers to all other learning tools or information sources recommended by instructors or sought out by a student to use in support of their own learning. These materials include things like reference books, dictionaries, websites, or study aids that are not evaluated by the instructor. This category of material gives students the opportunity to use course concepts to build upon skills and abilities. Auxiliary content includes optional activities and assignments that emphasize communication skills, collaboration, research literacy, and critical thinking. Auxiliary content could include things like a tour of a lab, resource guide on the library website, or a journal club. Depending upon the quality of additional resource materials that students find on their own, there may be conflicting information. It is helpful for instructors to learn about supplemental resources that may be relevant for their course so that they can answer questions for students about suitability of materials.

Information Presentation

Presentations impart information, provide explanation, and give examples. A presentation can simply be the instructor talking while students listen or a talk that is accompanied by a visual aid. Handouts or copies of slides (PowerPoint, Prezi, Google Slides, Doodly, etc.) can highlight key ideas. Ad hoc visuals, like writing on a white board or drawing a picture, can present an in-the-moment connection. Any visual aid in a presentation reinforces content because students see something as well as hear something in the lecture. Taking notes while listening to a lecture can help students pay attention and retain information: note taking is a kinesthetic activity.

In a live online presentation it is very difficult to keep attention of the audience especially when the presentation contains new information or material. If students are visible to the presenter and have the opportunity to ask questions, they can be more engaged in the lecture. For large groups of students, live questions can be chaotic if not managed well. Lengthy presentations to large groups lack the opportunity for interaction making it difficult for students to follow along. In a live lecture, the presenter can read the room to see when students get tired, restless, or look confused. It is more difficult to do this online.

Short presentations that are interspersed with other learning activities are more easily digestible for distance learning. After viewing a live presentation, students can break up into small groups for active learning exercises. Then, they return to the full class for a review and debriefing. This approach creates a learning arc that gives instructors time to share information and students a place, space, and time to delve more deeply to explore or apply concepts, then give feedback about what they learned.

Presentations can also be recorded for asynchronous viewing to allow students to watch and listen at their own pace. Lengthy lectures can be broken up into a series of shorter micro-lectures. This creates a natural opportunity for interleaving while students are studying. They can listen to a micro-lecture, read, complete an assignment for a different class, and then move on to the next micro-lecture. The interwoven activities help students retain information and ideas. Using shorter lectures also makes it easy for students to identify topics and find material to rewind for a second listen. Often prerecorded course lectures are used for flipped classrooms.

Lectures and presentations can be recorded several different ways using different technologies. Presentation capture apps (Camtasia, Panopto, Screenflow, or LMS integrations) offer the option to record a video of the screen along with an audio and video recording of the presenter from a webcam. Screen share videos with accompanying audio only are another option. For students with limited internet capabilities, MP3 audio recordings (Audacity, Adobe Audition) can be made to accompany downloadable PDFs of presentation slides. Because this approach requires less internet bandwidth it may be a more equitable way to deliver presentations so they are accessible to all students.

Other media including videos, television shows, or films can take the place of presentations. Professional organizations and **open education resources** are good places to look for material. Viewing a presentation by someone other than the course instructor can give students the experience of having a guest lecturer. When prerecorded media will be used for presentation, the instructional format would be different in distance learning compared to a face-to-face class. Whereas in a face-to-face session the class could view the media as a group and then discuss, a flipped classroom approach would work better in distance learning. Having the students view the media prior to class would maximize the potential for interaction during live meetings.

Readings

Readings are another way to present information. Typical readings in higher education include textbooks, book chapters, or journal articles. Other options for course readings include news reports, historical items, firsthand accounts, relevant blogs, etc. Readings can support, reinforce, or complement information from a video or audio presentation—or vice versa. Reading material should not be so complicated that it needs to be explained in a lecture.

Selection of reading material begins with the goals of the course and general abilities of the students. A course that has prerequisites can draw upon more challenging reading material than an introductory course. A creative mix of course readings can meet the needs of diverse learners and encourage information literacy. Fair use guidelines should be followed for all copyrighted materials.

When students are required to complete readings before a class session, the focus of the class can be using the readings. Class activities can explore and apply information from the reading. Students can have the opportunity to ask questions or seek clarifications about material covered in the readings.

To select readings, start by gathering textbooks used in previous offerings of the course. Look to see which textbooks have new editions and what content has been added or updated to provide insight into new information that needs to be emphasized. Next review other textbooks to compare and contrast material and presentation. For all textbooks under consideration explore the publisher's digital assets to find possible activities that can be incorporated into class. If price is a consideration, look for open educational resource textbooks or other readings. Review the content to ensure it provides adequate coverage of the topic. If a school or program publishes a booklist for students, review that list. Ensure that potential textbooks are on the list. If not, and a textbook looks like a good choice, recommend that it be added to the booklist.

For research and professional journal articles, review the list of articles previously used as required or recommended reading. Conduct a few searches to see whether there are more recent publications that might provide updated information. Consider articles that have been used previously and contrast the topic with the textbook. This can identify whether an article filled a gap or reinforced information. To avoid overloading students with work, curate the reading list by removing articles as new ones are added. Once the instructor has a preliminary reading list, the instructor should audit the content to ensure that topics are adequately covered without excessive duplication. To further narrow down the reading list, instructors should time readings to gauge the amount of time students will need to read during the course.

To identify potential source material for supplemental reading, it can be helpful to look back at previous terms to see sources suggested by students. As the final reading list is selected, the instructor should confirm that all reading material will be accessible during the course. That includes making sure that current editions of books are available, library resources can be placed on reserve (where applicable), and copyrighted materials are properly handled. If news reports, historical items, firsthand accounts, or blogs will be used for required, recommended, or supplemental reading, test to ensure that any hyperlinks are stable.

Intellectual Property

Questions about copyrights and use of material are often ask in the distance learning environment. Rights to materials is applicable both to materials selected for use in a course and materials created by instructors for teaching and learning. Intellectual property that is subject to copyright includes books, works of art, music, plays, poems, software, and images. It applies to materials such as manuals, workbooks, or forms that have been created for teaching and learning purposes.

Fair Use Doctrine

Fair use doctrine provides guidelines for the protection and distribution of copyrighted material. A copyright is exclusive legal right to material. It protects author(s) from repurposing, copying, or using material without permission. Textbooks, chapters, articles published in professional or peer reviewed journals, and other materials used in education are likely subject to copyright laws. Permission from authors is not necessarily required depending upon how the material is used. Fair use is a legal concept that allows limited use of copyrighted materials for educational purposes. In order for instructors to use copyrighted materials in a class, four basic criteria are applied.

- *Purpose* for the material. Fair use for educational purposes means that the copyrighted material should be used in class for instruction only and not commercial purposes.

- *Nature* of the copyrighted material. This refers to the material as a creative work, factual work, and even copyrighted work that is unpublished.

- The *amount* of the material used. When the entirety of the copyrighted material is not relevant to the course, educators should only use what is necessary for educational purposes. Examples of this would be a chapter from a book (instead of the whole book) or a single article from a peer reviewed journal (instead of the entire issue in which the article was published in the journal.)

- Potential result of or *effect* from use. There are some situations where use of copyrighted material could potentially harm the market for the selected materials. An example of this would be a workbook used in a program that the author of the workbook intends to publish for retail sale. If contents from the workbook were copied or given to students it would not be compliant with fair use.

The author(s) of the copyrighted material should receive attribution for any material used in a course. This means ensuring that the author(s) name(s) appear on copied documents, chapters, forms, or articles in their original form. In cases where the name is not on the material (e.g. a section or portion is abstracted) a reference or citation should be provided to give credit to the author(s). Compliance with fair use doctrine is voluntary—and ethical. Demonstrating compliance with fair use can be good modeling for students.

First Sale Doctrine

Institutional libraries purchase textbooks, subscribe to professional and academic journals, and buy other materials to create a pool of resources for use in teaching and learning. First sale doctrine is a legal concept that gives someone who has purchased copyrighted material the right to lend, share, or sell it without the obtaining permission of the owner of the copyright. Under first sale doctrine, libraries are required to control access to and limit use of materials, including digital resources to comply with intellectual property laws.

A library can lend books, digital media, and other copyrighted materials for educational purposes. However, the copyrighted material must be lent, shared, or sold in its original form. It cannot be copied, nor can a portion of it be copied or extracted. It is important to note that the language used to describe first sale doctrine generally describes institutions and organizations. But the legal concept is applicable to individuals including those who run workshops or collaborate on research and scholarly projects. An instructor who purchased a copyrighted item could lend it to a student. But the lending would need to have a specific purpose and be in a limited capacity. An example would be if a student was working on a scholarly project that involved research on a book that was in the instructor's personal collection. In this case the instructor could lend the book to the student.

Branded Materials

Some exercise science and kinesiology programs use branded course materials. Many programs that educate personal trainers or fitness instructors rely on branded course materials to educate students in how to structure a session or class. Slide decks, textbooks, videos, photographs, and other bespoke materials developed by and branded for a program are subject to intellectual property laws. These types of materials are intended for use intact. No portions should be extracted or copied for external use. Materials should not be altered without permission of the program or institution. A training program can purchase a license to use copyrighted and branded material. The terms of such arrangements are outlined in a licensing agreement.

Open Educational Resources

Open educational resources are freely accessible materials for use in teaching and learning. Original teaching materials are published in repositories under open licenses allowing educators to legally revise, reuse, retain, and redistribute materials. These include textbooks, courses, modules, recordings, and other materials in public domain or published under open license or creative commons license.

The intent behind open educational resources is to create information repositories as broad reservoirs of knowledge. Making materials freely accessible promotes equitable access by eliminating cost as a barrier. There is a worldwide open educational resources community comprised of different entities and interest groups that catalogue materials including OER Global, OER Commons, and Open Edition Books. Open educational resources promote innovation when educators modify and enhance materials and share them amongst themselves. Educators can be inspired by the way materials are revised, remixed, and how they are used. Educators who participate in open education resource movement must both extract and contribute materials in order for the concept to work.

Creating Materials

Instructors often create original materials for use in teaching and learning. When course materials have been prepared as part of one's job, the material is generally considered to be property of the institution. An instructor who desires to package and sell course materials developed as part of employment may not necessarily be able to do so without informing the institution and obtaining permission.

It is not customary for an instructor who is an employee of an institution to copyright manuals, workbooks, or slide presentations. Commercializing course content for payment or royalties can be considered a conflict of interest. If students are required to purchase the instructor's materials to use in class the instructor may benefit financially.

Instructors who choose to develop their own course materials and seek to commercialize them in some way should seek guidance from administration. The extent to which the instructor used release time and institutional resources to develop materials, along with how they used the materials in a course (allowing them to obtain feedback from students) effects who owns a copyright and/or is entitled to royalties.

Assignments

Assignments are tasks given to students that require them to engage with course material. Assignments teach students to work independently or collaboratively, follow directions, find and use resources, and meet deadlines. Assignments can be structured to help students dive deeper into concepts, review material, and practice skills. Assignments that are turned into the instructor for grading serve as assessments. A more creative way to leverage assignments is to use them as material for in-class activities. This is more easily accomplished with technology used in distance learning than in face-to-face classes. Assignments can be turned into teaching materials by using them in discussion forums. When students have the opportunity to revise, update, or augment an assignment after gaining insights from class discussion it promotes critical thinking.

Supplies

Regardless of instructional format, there are basic supplies students needed for a course. Something to use for note taking: a spiral notebook, notepad, loose leaf paper in a binder, or index cards and pen/pencil. Students may need a highlighter or adhesive page markers to mark important references. Paper clips, staples, and a stapler are needed to group items together. A binder, folders, or folio is helpful to organize notes and handouts. After the end of the course, the student can archive hard copies of materials for future reference.

Technology is a supply needed for distance learning. Students and instructors involved in distance learning will need to ensure that they meet technology requirements prior to enrollment in a program or course. Although most LMSs can be accessed on a smartphone or tablet, those types of devices lack some of the features necessary for engagement in a course. Technology supplies generally include:

- A basic functional set up is a computer, keyboard, pointing device (mouse or touchpad), webcam, microphone, and headset.

Using a headset instead of built in speakers and microphone will minimize audio feedback. Tablets can be adapted for use as a computer. However not all apps work on a tablet; some work differently or in a diminished capacity.

- Adequate storage space on the computer, an external or flash drive, or cloud-based storage to download and save course materials.

- Reliable high speed internet access. It is worth noting when students live with family or roommates that there may be competition for internet when others are studying or working from home. Course planning should consider this possibility and identify alternatives for students who have schedule conflicts or problems with logistics.

- Apps to access course files (e.g. PDF reader, Microsoft Office, Google Apps, media player.)

- Apps to produce documents (Word, Google Docs), slides (PowerPoint, Google Slides), spreadsheets (Excel, Google Sheets) or other types of files, and video/audio recordings.

- Software to take notes directly in electronic files (e.g. Notability, Acrobat Pro) can be useful for students who prefer electronic versions of course files.

In exercise science and personal training education, supplies to support teaching and learning include skeletons, muscle models, bands or markers to trace muscles. Student practice requires adequate space to practice with a safe surface, appropriate footwear, and a mat. If students in distance learning will be expected to practice or demonstrate exercises, equipment like weights, bands, stationary bicycle, plyo box, etc. will be needed. Students learning to perform tests would need equipment like a sit and reach box or yardstick, tape measure, stopwatch, blood pressure monitor, etc. as well as a person to practice with to perform assessments. Fitness testing equipment used at home during distance learning would not meet calibration standards for a laboratory but may be adequate for instructional purposes.

Course Planning

Planning a new course or revising an existing course can feel like putting together a puzzle. For distance learning, all course activities—including class meetings and assignments—need to fit into the instructional time and credit hours and flow in a logical manner. Materials and activities need to align with learning objectives for each session and for the course as a whole.

Instructional Time

Instructional activities include time spent in teaching and learning activities as well as self-directed activities (for students) and preparation/grading time (for instructors.) A course "hour" is generally 50 minutes of participation; however some schools use a 60 minute hour to calculate course credit. The full time equivalent (FTE) formula is used to calculate the number of credits a student takes to achieve full-time or part-time status. FTE is also used to calculate instructor workload. Lectures, labs, and clinical courses have different requirements for work performed in class and outside of class. Student course load and instructor workload take these calculations into account in attempts to ensure that time required for teaching and learning is manageable.

BEYOND LECTURES

Credit and Contact Hours

Undergraduate course credits are traditionally calculated based upon a combination of contact hours (when students and instructors are interacting live) and out-of-class student work (reading, writing papers, and completing assignments or projects.) The amount of time that individual students devote to out-of-class work can differ depending upon a student's academic preparedness, motivation, and effort. Students who are able to complete out-of-class work quickly will spend less time on a course compared to students who require more time to read or complete assignments. The time spent in class would be the same for all students who met attendance requirements regardless of who took more or less time.

A 15-week lecture course that meets for 3 hours each week would have additional work expected of students. Typically, this involves 2 hours of out-of-class work per credit hour for readings, homework, assignments, reviews, and studying. For the full term, the 3-credit course would be a total of 135 instructional hours. The lectures would provide 45 contact hours and the additional work would involve 90 total hours of instructional time.

Credit for laboratory and practicum courses is calculated using a ratio of 1 credit to 3 hours of participation time. This assumes that all instructional activity takes place in the lab or practicum and there is no out-of-class work required of students. Laboratory or practicum courses are all contact hours. So a 2 credit laboratory course would involve 6 contact hours per week for 15 weeks for a total of 90 hours of instructional time.

Distance learning courses calculate credits based upon the same formula. However, the credit hour calculation bears scrutiny because it does not simply refer to time spent logged into a learning management system. Course hours are calculated based upon all learning and instructional activities: viewing lectures, participating in discussions, and completing out-of-class assignments. A 3-credit course that ran for 15 weeks would still have a total of 135 instructional hours regardless of whether it involved live lectures or interactive sessions between students and instructors.

For undergraduate students, 12-15 credits is considered full time enrollment. This is the equivalent of 36-45 hours per week of total time spent on instructional activities. Being enrolled full time is basically the same as being employed full time in terms of hours.

Auditing Instructional Time

Instructors should avoid trying to accomplish too much in a course. Students should have adequate time to ask questions and complete assignments. Any reading or assignment that takes an excessive amount of time to complete may need to be revised or accounted for by balancing other independent work to ensure students are not overloaded. A guideline for creating out-of-class or independent work is to assume that any assignment or reading would take a student three times longer to complete than the instructor. For new instructors, timing themselves reading a chapter or completing an assignment can be useful to calculate how long an activity could take an average student. As instructors gain experience in curriculum development and teaching it becomes easier to estimate the amount of time a typical student will spend on an activity. Asking students how much time is spent on an assignment can provide more accurate insight to allocate instructional time for assignments in relation to overall coursework. This can be useful to ensure credit, contact hours, and workload are in balance; when necessary, adjustments can be made.

When a course is being planned, or in preparation for a new term, all instructional materials and activities should be reviewed against credit hours and contact hours for the course. Make a chart of all materials and activities for the course—including live class meetings. List the amount of time involved for each. Estimate the amount of time needed to complete each reading and assignment—then multiply by 3 for the time it will take an average student. Totaling the time for required readings provides an overview for the amount of time students will devote to that part of the course.

Instructor Workload

The time instructors spend teaching includes contact hours spent with students, preparation time, and grading assessments and assignments. At many undergraduate institutions 12 teaching credits is considered full-time. Working from the assumption that instructors spend two hours of time preparing for one teaching hour, a 12-credit teaching load equals a 36-hour workweek. This leaves 4 hours a week for instructors to contribute some of their time to institutional service and advisement of students in a 40-hour week.

At many institutions instructors who are full-time faculty do not work year-round. If research and scholarly activities are expected, that can be accounted for by not having teaching responsibilities in a summer session or winter term. For institutions that do not require research or scholarly activities, a heavier teaching load may be required during teaching semesters for full-time faculty who have summer or winter terms off. Depending upon where an exercise science, fitness, or kinesiology program is housed, faculty may be expected to engage in research and scholarly work. It may be needed for reappointment and promotion. When this is the case, time may be factored into workload for junior faculty.

Release Time

For new instructors, more time is typically needed to develop teaching materials and activities. Release time may or may not be granted in the first few years of a faculty member's appointment. This is essentially a reduced teaching load to allow time for course preparation. Once an instructor has a relatively stable course workload the extra preparation time is not expected to be necessary.

In higher education, full-time faculty who are expected to be scholars in their discipline may negotiate release time for research, writing, or creative activities. For new full-time faculty this is generally negotiated based upon teaching credits. The instructor is expected to produce something (e.g. research study, manuscript) as a result of the time released from teaching. Instructors may apply for grant funding to cover costs of research or a scholarly project. Funds from the grant may be applied to release time effectively covering the cost of hiring a temporary instructor as replacement to teach.

For instructors in exercise science and personal training, staying up-to-date with the profession is essential. This includes continuing education and other requirements to renew professional licenses and certifications. Institutions do not generally grant release time for these purposes. But it adds to the overall workload for instructors.

Part-Time Faculty

Throughout higher education, part-time faculty are hired to teach on a contract basis. Historically, these types of positions were filled by individuals who brought specialized expertise and real-world experience to add depth to academic departments. In recent decades, a larger percentage of higher education faculty appointments were part-time. While the experts are still hired to fill those positions, the teaching contracts often allow very little time for course preparation. This can cause work to be front-loaded which can be overwhelming.

There is generally no expectation for adjunct faculty to engage in research or scholarly activities. Adjunct faculty may be given access to the library to use for research if they choose. If they opt to do so, it is on their own time and does not factor into their part-time workload.

Class Schedule

An appeal of distance learning is flexibility. But there is still a need to structure participation in class activities to ensure students are engaged and have adequate time to complete activities. Transparency about the class schedule is very important. For synchronous courses prospective students should be informed prior to enrollment about the class meeting schedule so they can make the decision to register—or not. Jobs, caregiving, personal and family responsibilities can interfere with ability to attend class sessions. All distance learning courses, regardless of format, should provide information about the amount of time expected each week to participate in class activities to help students plan.

Course Policies

Course policies outline requirements for successful completion of coursework as well as expectations for student behavior and participation. Some policies are at the discretion of the course instructor while others may be required by the institution. When planning a course, instructors should consider how polices will promote learning and also how policies can be enforced if/when they are violated.

A policy for attendance and participation requires a method of measurement such as students being visible on a webcam during a live course session, logging into the LMS, or contributing to a discussion forum. Instructions for assignments should include policies regarding incomplete work or assignments turned in late. Requirements for make-up activities should be outlined for students who miss a class or fall short of participation requirements.

Accessibility and Accommodations

Federal law requires that a person with a disability has the same opportunity to learn and participate fully in a course as a person without a disability. All course materials and activities must be equally accessible to all students including those with physical disabilities or learning disabilities. Regardless of whether a course is offered online, face-to-face, or as a hybrid, adaptations may be needed to course materials or instructional strategies to meet needs of students with disabilities. These adaptations fall into a few basic categories: presentation, assessments, time, and environment.

Presentation

The way information is presented in a visual, auditory, or kinesthetic way should be accessible to all students or capable of adaptation if needed. Differentiated instruction is the presentation of the same material in multiple ways (e.g. video presentation and a transcript.) This provides all students with different options to engage with course material. That can be helpful for students who have different preferences for reading or listening. It can be useful to meet the needs of students with disabilities.

Principles from the Universal Design for Learning (UDL) provide a framework for accessibility in instructional design. These general ideas can be used in any course to benefit all students, not just students with disabilities. Some ways that courses can be made more accessible to all students include:

- Use video captions on presentations.

- Have a sign language interpreter for live or recorded presentations.

- Provide transcriptions of presentations and lectures.

- Record presentations so students can play back or review.

- Create documents and presentations using large print and/or high contrast.

- Attach descriptions to image files embedded in documents or presentations.

- Use black & white or gray scale instead of color on presentations and documents.

- Format documents for screen readers (e.g. structured headings, descriptive hyperlinks, and text descriptions of images.)

- Use consistent formatting for course documents and presentations.

During the development of a course instructional designers should plan for different ways to present information. For courses already in progress, documents, slides, and presentations can be formatted for alternate methods of delivery. Speech to text software can be used to create transcripts. Captions or subtitles can be selected in PowerPoint or Google Slides. It is relatively easy to convert a color presentation to black & white and/or to create large print versions of course documents.

Assessment and Time

Students demonstrate their knowledge, skills, and abilities by submitting assignments, taking tests, and completing assessments. Revision to what students are required to submit as well as procedures for assignments/tests/assessments may be needed to accommodate students with disabilities. Students may need extra time, have difficulty understanding instructions, or have challenges focusing, or may need to take breaks. Some general ways that courses can be made accessible include:

- Clearly outlined instructions and expectations for assignments.

- Offer options to submit assignments in written or recorded (audio or video) form.

- Offer students the option for informal review of assignments prior to final submission.

- Scaffold assignments to be completed in stages so students get feedback that they can use to improve the next stage for the assignment.

- Allow students unlimited time on tests or assessments.

- Configure online tests to allow saving of answers and student re-entry in case internet connection fails.

Students who have physical disabilities may need accommodations in labs that require exercise participation or demonstration of fitness tests. Instructors must take this into account when designing all learning activities.

Learning Environment

The need for accommodations varies depending upon whether a course is taught online, face-to-face, or as a hybrid. For the in-person component of any class, accommodations that might be needed include adaptive equipment, seating near the instructor, seating to alleviate discomfort, a note-taker, a sign language interpreter, or ability to take breaks. For testing and assessments a quiet space without distractions may be needed.

- Supply adaptive equipment for face-to-face classes.

- Offer the option for assigned seats in a face-to-face class.

- Provide different options for desks and seating.

- Contract with a note-taker or sign language interpreter when needed.

- Provide a dedicated proctored testing room.

When a course is designed with accessibility in mind it may minimize the need for a student to request accommodations. But if accommodations are necessary students and instructors should follow proper procedures regarding requests. This is important to protect the student's privacy and ensure that the accommodation does not reduce expectations or minimize what the student learns.

Course Structure

Because distance learning has multiple interpretations, consideration for the structure of a course is important. First a designation of the course as synchronous, asynchronous or hybrid must be made. Next the course goals, topics, and content should be arranged in a way that can facilitate student learning and communication among all course participants.

Effective and engaging methods used in teaching and learning for distance education are different than methods used in face-to-face classes. Effective distance learning requires strategies to connect instructors with students, foster connections among students, and promote self-directed learning. Lectures are part of instruction, but should not be the only instructional strategy if students are to be engaged in the learning process. Regardless of whether a lecture is delivered live or recorded, a lecture is a passive learning experience that relies on the student to make connections to course material. Facilitating instruction, not explaining information, engages students in the learning process.

When distance learning uses interaction, collaboration, and strategies for dialogue among students, it can be highly effective to promote learning. In distance learning this requires adaptations to methods of instruction and communication to draw students in, hear from them, and work with them. Distance learning can include passive activities to convey information. But effective distance learning also requires innovation and adaptation. Some material and people easily transition to distance learning formats. Others require more effort in order to learn and help students thrive.

Instructional Activities

Engaging distance learning is not simply instructors facing a gallery of students on webcams and imparting information for a scheduled period of time. It requires interaction between students and course material, the instructor, and each other. In order for a course to be engaging, some aspect of the time, place, and space of the learning experience may need to shift. Active learning and curated interactions require creativity to develop, but can substantially enhance retention of course material. Opportunities for informal discussion help students feel connected and explore ideas. Inclusion of low-stakes assessments helps monitor student progress and identify early needs for remediation. Moving away from a lecture-centric course does not mean doing away with lectures all together. Rather, strategic use of lectures for material that requires explanation opens up course time for facilitated learning opportunities.

Learning Arcs

For the entire course and every session, approaching instruction as a learning arc helps provide direction and promote cohesion. There are many ways educators can plan curriculum. A very basic way to think about it is a **learning arc** from introduction through exploration to review. The process of teaching and learning happens throughout the arc. When learning is a process, it is not sequential introduction and explanation of new material. Rather it is the opportunity for students to work with information.

A more robust example found in classical music. **Sonata allegro form** is a structure used in composition of a movement in a symphony: introduction, development, recapitulation. In the movement of a symphony, a theme is introduced, it is played with multiple variations, and then the theme is revisited including some of the variations. An instructional session can follow the same basic format.

- The *introduction* component is presentation of course material.

- The *development* aspect involves exploration, experimentation, clarification, and application.

- The *recapitulation* includes summarizing, review, or restatement of key information that was revealed during the development.

This sonata allegro form provides a framework to connect material throughout the session and provides an arc that guides the student through a learning experience. Each unit/module in distance learning can be viewed as its own learning arc. The introductory component is the presentation and explanation of material through lectures, readings, and assignments. This is used to prime students for exploration and application. The development component is where students and the instructor come together in active learning. Review, application, integration, and experimentation with material can happen during live online sessions or using asynchronous instructional activities. The recapitulation component can include a summary, review, and reflection. This might also include a follow up assignment that encourages students to apply material and concepts from the unit/module. An entire course can be designed to follow a learning arc from the beginning to the end.

Musculoskeletal anatomy provides a good example where learning arcs can be used to contextualize learning that is often explanatory. Students need to learn origins, insertions, and actions of muscles. This often involves memorization. Presenting this information in a live lecture can be dry and not very engaging. Requiring students to study muscle groups before class, then using class time to review and answer questions is a start. Students could then take turns exploring how the anatomy of muscles contributes to execution of typical joint movements. The application of information can help students remember the anatomy. To end class, a quick review of origins, insertions, and actions provides a summary that ends the learning arc for that session.

Using learning arcs in distance learning creates a flow. It offers opportunities for innovation, creativity, and ingenuity in virtual classrooms. The multiple opportunities for connection can promote a sense of belonging for students and help instructors get feedback on their progress.

Organizing Instructional Material

A course in an LMS can be designed different ways: in sequential order or with information clustered by topic. There should be a logical flow to show students where to look next in order to follow along. Organizing course activities in instructional units or modules helps students recognize how different learning activities fit together. To keep students from jumping ahead instructional material can be dripped: released when the unit/module is being taught. This helps students stay on track. Units/modules can remain open as the course progresses to encourage students to refer back to material as needed throughout the course.

An administrative section should be located at the top of the course page. This section should contain the syllabus, link to gradebook, and general announcements. An introductions forum can be placed here so it is easy for students to refer back to it as the course progresses. Information and a link or phone number to access the virtual classroom for live course meetings should be placed here—if the same method will be used for every synchronous session. However if this will change during the course, a new link for each meeting should be placed in the appropriate unit. This will ensure that students enter the correct virtual classroom for a synchronous session. The administrative section should be static at the top of the course page for easy access. It is the first place students look when they enter the virtual classroom.

Each unit/module should contain an overview or description of the material that will be covered. It may be helpful to include a brief review summarizing what students are expected to know and remember at that point in the course. All instructional activities for a unit/module should be provided in one place: presentations, slides, notes, handouts, discussion forums for that unit/module, and a place to submit assignments (if applicable.) All units/modules should have a consistent organization with topics, presentations, forums, assignments, activities, and external links posted in the same order for each unit/module. This helps to create a consistent flow within each unit/module and helps guide the student through activities.

Opening dates for each unit/module, and due dates for activities, should be clearly displayed for each unit/module. This is especially important when the unit/module will span an irregular length of time (e.g. two or three weeks, or less than one week.) Although flexibility is one of the most useful aspects of distance learning, flexibility can easily lead to disorganization. Sending reminders for due dates as course announcements or postings on a course calendar can help students stay on top of deadlines.

Parallel structure should be used to name and provide details for the same activity throughout the course. Example: Research Paper should always be referred to as Research Paper and not Research Project, Student Project, or term paper. Consistent naming helps to ensure students remember what the activity is, what they need to do and when. Consistent formatting for course documents and presentations helps students get oriented in the learning environment. All instructions and expectations for assignments should be clearly detailed.

Organization of instructional materials is the digital equivalent managing a face-to-face classroom session. A difference is that the organization in a virtual classroom needs to take place before the students arrive. As more instructors and students become familiar with the distance learning environment, course navigation will become easier for participants.

Instructional Strategies

Instructional strategies are techniques used in teaching to convey information to students and engage them in the learning process. Selection of instructional strategies in distance learning should aim to meet course goals and objectives while also keeping in mind availability of necessary tools and technologies. Instructional strategies can be placed into one of three broad categories: passive, active, and experiential.

Passive learning is delivery of course content for student consumption. The instructor is the subject matter expert who is responsible for imparting information to students who are expected to comprehend and use the information. Passive learning requires students to listen, read, and provide some type of evidence to indicate that they heard or read something. Lectures are an example of passive learning. The application of material from lectures occurs later in a test or assignment. Passive learning strategies are generally not engaging.

Active learning is learning that involves participation in an exercise, task, game, or assignment that uses course content. Students are required to do something. For successful active learning students need to take responsibility to participate. Bloom's Taxonomy can provide inspiration for active learning in the cognitive learning domain. Activities that allow students to show that they remember (know and comprehend), can use (apply, analyze) or practice (synthesize and evaluate) material demonstrates learning progression. This can take place in a single course or throughout an educational program.

Experiential learning is a form of active learning that involves a realistic scenario. David Kolb's experiential learning cycle is often used to outline a process in experiential learning. The four stages in the cycle are: concrete learning, reflective observation, abstract conceptualization, and active experimentation. Experiential learning relies on the assumption that students learn by doing. Inclusion of reflection and then repeating the cycle helps students experiment in the activity.

Distance learning in exercise science and personal training education can use instructional strategies in all of these categories to provide variety for students and balance to instructor workload. Using a combination of explanation and facilitation balances delivery of material with synchronous or asynchronous interaction when students have the opportunity to explore material, seek clarifications, and apply course concepts. Instructional strategies described in this section of the book can be selected to facilitate engagement with students for any type of class session.

Eight instructional strategies are presented in the next section of the book. Discussions, flipping the classroom, just in time instruction, case-based learning, team-based learning, project-based learning, problem-based learning, peer teaching, and observation/simulation. With the exception of team-based learning, all of the strategies can be implemented for an individual or small group format.

Although there are different interpretations of some instructional strategies among academic disciplines, active learning is a general concept that is highly adaptable. For each strategy presented, several examples are provided to show how they can be implemented in exercise science and personal training education. Included in the examples are opportunities for student engagement, interaction with instructors, information literacy, clinical reasoning, and collaboration.

Engaging Discussions

Discussions in distance learning can take place in live class sessions or asynchronously using discussion forums in the LMS. Depending on the size of the class, students can participate individually or in small groups. Instructions for each discussion should outline requirements for participation. Methods of assessment for discussions should be provided to all students before a live or online discussion begins. Discussions can be stand-alone assignments or woven into other instructional activities to provide opportunity for mutual feedback.

A discussion used as a stand-alone assignment starts with a prompt and instructions. The prompt should be a statement or question that is thought provoking and has a level of complexity. To promote interaction, there should be no single, obvious correct response or answer. Requiring answers to be connected to course materials can help ensure discussions stay focused. If contributions to the discussion are opinions, students should be required to support the opinion by citing course materials or other resources.

Using different **structures** for discussion contributions can help students pay attention to the conversation and make a quality contribution. The structures can be adapted for discussions held during live classes by allowing students time to prepare before the class meeting.

One option is to give students a **formula** to respond to other student's discussion answers. Ask them to include an acknowledgement, a detailed observation, and suggestion for further exploration or possible application of an idea.

Another formula has students taking turns being the **primary responder** to—and facilitator for—a discussion question. In large classes several students can be primary responders by submitting a response and facilitating one area of the conversation about the topic. This provides multiple opportunities for participation and can provide interesting variety in the answers.

A formula for responses to encourage engagement is the **3-part format**. An initial contribution is required by the first deadline (Part 1.) A response to two or more students (or other small groups) is required to meet the second deadline (Part 2.) A reflection or reaction is required to meet the third deadline (Part 3.) The 3-part format formula works well for asynchronous discussions that span a period of time (e.g. a week or course unit.) The 3-part format formula also works for small groups during live class sessions. The initial contribution can be a 1 to 2 minute report from each group on their ideas about the topic and list of resources they are using. The rest of the class can ask questions or make recommendations to meet a second deadline. Next the small groups continue their internal discussions to prepare an answer. Then all groups present a final 1 to 2 minute report on their findings by the third deadline.

To help facilitate synchronous or asynchronous discussions, assign students to small groups. Use the same group for a few class sessions before reconfiguring the groups. This allows students to get to know each other and can make it easier for instructors to track participation. It also helps to create balanced groups when achievement-oriented students are paired with students who are struggling. Creating groups comprised of 4 to 7 students can provide opportunities for all group members to participate.

For live class discussions organize the number of groups for the class to allow time for reporting from each group. A 2 minute report from 8 to 10 discussion groups in a live class will take approximately 30 minutes including time for questions from other students and feedback from the instructor. The report back from small groups is essential to ensure that groups work on the activity during the time allotted in class.

Begin the session with an overview and explicit instructions for the activity. Allow time for groups to get organized and engage with the topic. Have all groups report back to the class to make sure information is shared with the whole class. It can be convenient to break students into pairs or trios to share-and-compare. But students may not feel motivated to participate when there is no requirement for all pairs/trios to report back. Whenever possible, use small groups for discussions and include a deliverable (presented orally or in writing) to involve all students and maximize opportunities for engagement.

To organize small group activities, give students a list of roles they can use in their group. At minimum groups should have a manager/facilitator (to lead the discussion) and a recorder/reporter (to take notes and share findings with the class.) Additional roles can include: topic master (to make sure all parts of the discussion assignment are covered), researcher/runner (to get supporting information), consensus builder (to keep track of different opinions), and a timekeeper.

For evaluations of discussions, students should be able to say what role they filled for their group. Incorporate self-assessment in grading to encourage participation and reflection. For small group activities, require students to identify their role, primary contributions, and specify the percent effort their work contributed to the group as a whole. For individual discussions, ask students to rate the quality of their participation in the overall class discussion, resources used, the percent of their own contribution, and identify one new thing they learned in the discussion. Include the self-assessment grade as a portion of the student's grade for the discussion. Accountability can be an incentive to participate; especially important if students lack motivation.

Discussion Example 1

A live lecture on the pathophysiology of diabetes and the effects of exercise can be replaced with an activity that applies and synthesizes information. This can be done using small groups or having all students participate individually. It can be adapted for asynchronous discussion. The discussion and activities would be 9 hours of instructional time.

Prior to class, students complete assigned readings on diabetes. The instructor begins class with a brief presentation on pathophysiology of diabetes.

Small groups are assigned to review a complication that may occur in clients with diabetes (e.g. cardiovascular disease, neuropathy, kidney disease, retinopathy, skin conditions.) Small groups convene for 20 minutes to review course materials or other resources to use to create a bullet point summary of the complication.

The class comes back together and a designated reporter from each group shares their summary with the class.

After all presentations are finished, each group reconvenes to prepare a list of 5 questions on a health history form for a client with diabetes. The questions should seek a mix of general information about diabetes and specific information related to the complication and how that could factor into assessments and exercise program design. All groups post their list of questions to a collaborative document or wiki.

The class comes back together and the instructor leads a facilitated discussion on what information is important to know about clients with diabetes.

Discussion Example 2

This discussion could be live or asynchronous to replace a lecture on the cardiovascular system and cardiovascular disorders. The assigned readings and discussion activities would be 9 hours of instructional time.

Students prepare for class by completing assigned readings on the cardiovascular system and common cardiovascular disorders.

Class begins with a short presentation on hypertension.

Students break into small groups and search for statistics on prevalence of primary or secondary hypertension in different populations.

The class reconvenes and the reporter for each group summarizes what they found and where they found it.

The instructor then assigns each group to further research for information on what to consider in exercise for one type of hypertension. Each group looks for reference information and summarizes what they found in a discussion forum or wiki. Groups can then discuss how this information can be used in exercise program planning.

The class reconvenes and groups take turns presenting key insights for their assigned condition.

The instructor concludes the session with a short summary of research findings on the effects of exercise on blood pressure.

Discussion Example 3

A lecture on musculoskeletal disorders can be replaced with an interactive session that uses a short lecture as a summary. This is described as a small group activity but could be adapted for individual student participation. The reading, preparation, and discussion could be configured to be 6 hours of instructional time.

To prepare for class students would be required to read a textbook chapter.

Class begins with an introduction to the activity.

Small groups are assigned two musculoskeletal disorders to compare and contrast. Examples: hamstring strain/iliotibial band syndrome, meniscus tear/patellofemoral syndrome, and thoracic outlet syndrome/whiplash. Each group should have different conditions to allow coverage of multiple conditions in the session.

Working in small groups, students identify 3 activities or occupations associated with risk for the disorders (e.g. meniscus tear/patellofemoral syndrome in warehouse workers, firefighters, soccer players.) Each small group should write their response in a discussion forum in the LMS that is accessible to the entire class.

The class comes back together and a designated reporter from each group briefly summarizes the disorders and occupations/activities on their list. After all groups have reported, the information is passed to a new group.

Each small group now has a new disorder and a list of occupations/activities. All groups are tasked with investigating approaches that are used to reduce risk of the musculoskeletal disorders in the occupations/activities on their list. This can be summarized in the discussion forum including citations for the source of the information.

The class comes back together. A designated reporter from each group can share one risk reducing approach (e.g. active warm ups used in soccer.) After all groups have reported, the instructor can end class with a brief presentation on ways to reduce risk for common musculoskeletal disorders.

Flipped Classroom

The flipped classroom model requires students to complete work prior to class (pre-work) leaving class time to be used for discussions, questions, and activities. An easy way to conceptualize a flipped classroom is to think about it like a lab. The activities, experiences, or experiments help students apply and synthesize course material.

To conceptualize a flipped classroom, view the full learning experience as an arc:

- The pre-work introduces course material.
- The discussion or activity reinforces or explores concepts or ideas.
- Something is produced that builds upon the pre-work and experimentation or discussion.

The learning arc formed in a flipped classroom can guide the student through the process from introduction through application of the material. There are many forms of pre-work. Students can listen to prerecorded lectures or podcasts, read chapters, books, or articles or complete assignments. It is essential that the pre-work is utilized in some way during the class session.

A low stakes assessment (a short quiz or assignment) can be used as evidence that students completed the pre-work. When work is completed during class, it produces something that can be used as another low stakes assessment. Students could present results of their work to the class for another assessment. It is essential to make the pre-work highly relevant to the course discussion or in class activities to entice students to do the required work before class.

The challenge in a flipped classroom model is that it requires student participation. When students do not participate, it contributes to one of two types of problems.

> Students do not complete the pre-work. When they do not arrive to class prepared, they lack information. It can be difficult to engage them when they are trying to make up work.

or

> Students do not fully participate during the class meeting. This can happen when they are used to passive learning. It is also common if students fail to recognize value of the activity or the activity is confusing.

Planning and preparation are vital to make a flipped classroom effective. Careful organization with clear directions and learning outcomes can help create successful sessions. Preparing students for what to expect is essential. A flipped classroom takes a little imagination, but the result is an experience that is more engaging than a lecture.

Flipped Classroom Example 1

In place of a live lecture on pathophysiology of the cardiovascular system a flipped classroom approach could be used.

Pre-work: Assigned reading in textbook. Students listen to a prerecorded lecture that includes video on cardiovascular circulation.

Assignment: List 5 key points that are important to know about risk for cardiovascular disorders. All students submit their lists to instructor prior to class session. Prior to class (or while the students are working in class) the instructor can sort the lists from each student to identify key points that students believe are important.

Class Session: Students work in small groups for 10 minutes to choose one key point or risk factor from their compiled lists to review with the class. Students submit their selected key point to the LMS discussion forum. If key points are duplicated, the instructor can ask groups to select a new point to enable each group to have an individual topic.

Each group prepares a mini-lecture (3 to 5 minutes) to review that key point. This could be in the form of a written summary with bullet points or a few slides. Each group shares the materials for their mini lecture to the LMS.

Next one member from each group presents the mini-lecture to the class.

The instructor can summarize any key points that were overlooked by the class to give students an opportunity to review.

Assessments: Each student's list of key points, the group's summary and presentation.

Flipped Classroom Example 2

This activity could replace a lecture in a unit/module in anatomy & physiology on the peripheral nervous system. Organizing the class into no more than 5 groups would allow time for the activity in a 3 hour live class session.

Pre-work: Students read a chapter in the textbook on the nervous system.

Assignment: All students submit a list prior to class of three concepts that they understand clearly (e.g. somatic nervous system, neuron anatomy, myelin) and three concepts for which they need clarification or explanation (e.g. interneurons, dermatomes, nociception.)

Prior to class (or while the students are working in class) the instructor can review lists from each student to identify common topics that need clarification or explanation.

Class Session: Students are assigned to small groups to prepare bullet points to explain one concept that they understand clearly. A member from each group presents their summary to the class.

Next each group tackles a concept for which they need more explanation. They summarize what they know. A member of the group presents to the class. Other groups—or the instructor—can offer to fill in missing information to help the group understand the concepts.

To conclude the class, the instructor can summarize topics the class understands already and present bullet points from topics that a majority of the students need clarified or explained. This can help students identify material to review in the textbook or from supplementary course resources.

Assessments: Each student's list of concepts, the group's summary and presentation.

Flipped Classroom Example 3

This activity could replace a structured review for a summative assessment or a live question and answer session. Review of material is included at three different steps: before the session (in pre-work and the assignment), during the session (while producing material in the group study guide) and during the review of the different group study guides.

Pre-work: Each student creates a study guide to review materials to for the upcoming exam. The study guide is uploaded as an assignment to the LMS.

Assignment: Prior to class, students take a brief online quiz. The quiz is automatically graded so students receive immediate feedback.

Class Session: The instructor gives general feedback on the quiz performance. Students are then sorted into small groups based upon their quiz score. Each group should contain a mix of quiz scores.

Working in groups, students collaborate to produce a new study guide. They can take turns sharing their individual study guides to compare what information is included, how it is presented, and discuss whether it is easy to use—or not.

Next the groups share their study guides with the rest of the class. A reporter for each group can summarize the process and the structure of the study guide.

The instructor—or students in other groups—can give feedback on contents and different formats.

Assessments: Each student's quiz score, each student's individually prepared study guide, and the group's study guide.

Just in Time Instruction

Just in Time teaching is a flipped classroom approach that uses assessments to tailor teaching activities. It provides a more engaging approach than an explanatory lecture because students arrive in a class session with some familiarity about the topic. Assessments are used both as an incentive for students to prepare for class and to help instructors identify material that needs additional presentation or exploration. In-class time can be used more efficiently by paying less attention to material students understand well and focusing on topics that students find complex or complicated.

Just in Time begins with a self-directed study activity. Generally, this is reading a textbook chapter. But it could also involve watching a prerecorded lecture, reading a journal article, or accessing another informational resource.

Once the self-directed activity is completed, students are required to complete an assessment. This can be a short quiz or an assignment. Using quizzes helps students become more practiced at test taking strategies. Textbook ancillary materials (worksheets, games, puzzles, reviews of videos) can work well in this instructional strategy. It can also be helpful to show students how to utilize a range of different types of materials to support their learning.

Students submit the assessment for grading 24 to 48 hours before the class session.

The instructor reviews the assessment results to identify topics that are in most need of clarification or explanation.

The class session can be tailored by the instructor to center around the material that requires clarification, explanation, or exploration. It should also include acknowledgement of material that the majority of the students know well. This type of reinforcement can help students recognize how to structure their own study time efficiently.

This type of instruction does put a last-minute burden on instructor. It requires flexibility and a quick turnaround to adapt class activities to targeted material. But it can be a useful to provide ongoing assessment. It can also be helpful for courses that have a large amount of content to cover in a short amount of time because it teaches students to be self-directed learners.

Just in Time Instruction Example 1

This activity could replace a full session lecture on the endocrine system by targeting material that is in most need of explanation or review.

For a unit/module in anatomy & physiology on the endocrine system, students read a textbook chapter. At least 48 hours before the class session they take a 10-question quiz on the chapter.

The instructor reviews the quiz grades and prepares a short presentation to review material from questions that received the lowest scores. This allows the instructor to source material from a larger endocrine system lecture and use only a portion to present material in need of review or clarification.

Next an online poll can be used to have the whole class complete a second 8 to 10 question quiz during the class session in real time. This quiz should have more complex questions and possible answers that require careful consideration. After students record their answer to a question, the answer distribution can be revealed. Next students can share their thought process used to arrive at their answer. The class can defend or debate the answers. After discussion the instructor can summarize key information and then reveal the correct answer before moving on to the next question.

A challenge that can occur when using polling and discussion is over-sharing by eager students. If this occurs, students can be allowed to only speak up once. Another challenge is students who are reluctant to speak up (often because they are afraid of being wrong.) They can be asked to describe one step in their thought process, or share what materials they used to arrive at an answer. This will include them as part of the discussion without making them uncomfortable.

Just in Time Instruction Example 2

This activity could replace an anatomy & physiology lecture that describes origins, insertions, and actions of muscles. This type of activity can be helpful for any content that requires memorization. Instead of presenting the information, students review multiple times and engage in assessments.

Prior to a class on musculoskeletal anatomy students can complete a matching or labeling worksheet with origins, insertions, and actions of muscles of one area of the body (e.g. the hip joint.) Students can mark any answers for which they are uncertain or would like more clarification. Students scan and submit their completed worksheets as an assignment.

The instructor reviews and grades the answers. At the beginning of class the instructor can prepare a short presentation that focuses on incorrect answers and requests for clarification. The lecture can be oriented toward anatomical landmarks and characteristics of muscles that help give insight into their actions. This could involve topics like contrasting the location and actions of the gluteal muscles, comparing different actions of the anterior hip muscles, or reviewing the location of the psoas muscles.

Students can then work in groups to prepare a list of activities that concentrically contract different hip muscles to produce movements. The lists can be shared with the class and/or submitted as another assessment for grading.

Just in Time Instruction Example 3

This activity could replace a lecture describing joint movements and muscle actions. Review and experimentation help students have a visual and kinesthetic experience while identifying concepts that are challenging.

For a kinesiology unit/module students prepare for class students by viewing a movement video that demonstrates complex movement sequences (e.g. baseball pitch, weightlifter performing a clean & press, ballerina pirouette.)

The assessment is a worksheet that students complete analyzing the actions of muscles that produce specific movement in the video.

Prior to class, the instructor reviews the worksheet answers to identify collective areas of weakness. Then the instructor prepares a short lecture clarifying muscle actions in relation to the video movements and other movements.

Students then break into small groups to identify other activities that use the muscles in a similar way. Each group prepares a list of 2 to 3 activities and lists the muscles. Then groups report back to the class to summarize their findings.

To conclude the class the instructor can summarize similarities and differences among the selected activities.

Case-Based Learning

Case-based learning involves application of course content to a client scenario. Case-based instruction promotes critical thinking and provides a safe place for students to practice applying and integrating course material. Because there is no single right answer for a case it can make students nervous. This is especially applicable to high achieving students who set their sights on good grades. Using case scenarios during class and for assignments may nudge these types of students away from a focus on achievement towards listening and learning about clients. For students who are slower learners, taking time to work through a case can help them review, apply concepts, and self-assess their knowledge in a low stakes environment. Case-based activities can be used as a break out section in a lecture course by having students work individually or in small groups and then present information to the class.

Exercise science, kinesiology, personal training, and fitness typically uses labs or peer teaching for active learning. But there are many more possibilities for instruction, especially to help students develop critical thinking skills. Working with a case scenario would not take the place of a lab session. But it does present an opportunity for review, application of concepts, and integration of information needed to make decisions about selection of assessments or exercise program design.

If didactic and theory-based courses are distinct from labs or peer teaching, it can be difficult for students to integrate information and apply concepts. This is a known gap throughout clinical education. A student might learn the pathophysiology of Type 2 diabetes in a lecture and design an exercise program as part of a lab session. Putting the two together is essential. Case-based learning provides an opportunity to bridge the gap by engaging students in active learning using a cognitive approach. Interactive discussion, brainstorming, research-based assignments, and treatment planning can all be used to apply concepts and reinforce learning.

Case-based learning works well in both face-to-face classrooms and virtual classrooms for either synchronous or asynchronous classes. Case-based assignments can be used as low stakes assessments. To minimize burden of grading for the instructor, student work can be used as material for in-class activities. A flipped classroom approach works well with case-based learning. Students can review cases prior to class and complete assignments to prepare them to use the case in class for learning activities.

Case-Based Learning Example 1

This activity could replace a lecture on disorders of the knee in pathophysiology or a presentation on client interviewing.

Provide the students with paragraph presenting a narrative of a case scenario. It can be written on a slide that is shared on the computer and projected to a screen or on a document posted to the LMS. For example:

> 57 year old investment banker who loves to play tennis. He plays several times a week for fitness and for networking. He strained the medial collateral ligament in his right knee several years ago while skiing. Completed physical therapy treatments and still does leg strengthening exercises on a regular basis. Recently he was diagnosed with osteoarthritis of the knee. He is currently wearing a knee brace on his right knee when he plays tennis to prevent hyperextension.

Give students time to read through the case scenario and underline or list keywords or information that would be relevant to a health history interview.

Bring the class together to review the scenario as a group. Have students take turns identifying different keywords in the case that they think are important. Ask them to provide rationale.

Once all important keywords have been identified, the instructor can summarize the information for the class and illustrate where the relevant information should be noted on a health history form.

Case-Based Learning Example 2

This activity could replace a pathophysiology lecture or a presentation on client interviewing.

Sort the students into small groups and give each group a different case scenario. The scenario can be a written narrative or a health history form prepared as if it has been completed by a client.

Working in their groups, the students make a list of questions to ask the client for clarification or to obtain additional information that might be relevant to a sign, symptom, medical diagnosis, or health-related behavior.

Next, each group presents their case scenario to the class. They share their list of questions. Other groups can ask for rationale behind questions or make suggestions for additional information that might be needed from the client.

To encourage participation by all students, assign roles to each group member (e.g. facilitator, recorder, reporter, and timekeeper.) At the conclusion of the activity, invite one student from different groups who performed the same assigned role to summarize how they contributed to the work of their group.

As students become more practiced at working with case-based learning, less time will be needed. The discussion can take place in 15 to 20 minutes. So this type of activity can be used in a class session after a lecture or 2 or 3 rounds of this type of activity can be completed over a full class session.

Case-Based Learning Example 3

This activity could replace a lecture in kinesiology or pathophysiology that covers movement dysfunction.

With students working in small groups, assign each group a different case scenario that involves movement dysfunction or limited range of motion. The format could include several conditions that affect the same area of the body (e.g. rotator cuff injury, separated shoulder, torn biceps, thoracic outlet syndrome) to help students compare and contrast disordered movements.

Each group reviews their case with the goal of creating a biopsychosocial assessments protocol. The goal would be to gather information on the holistic impact of the movement dysfunction or limited range of motion. The assessment list could include active and passive range of motion tests, questions or scales that explore how the limitation affects mood/mental state, and the extent to which the limitation could affect work and social activities.

The class can reconvene and each group can summarize their case and report descriptions of their selected assessments with the class.

After all groups have reported, the class can compare and contrast different assessment approaches.

Team-Based Learning

Team-based learning is structured small group learning where each member of the team is accountable to the others in contribution to a single answer. This involves collaboration, critical thinking, discourse, persuasion, and negotiation. Team-based learning requires individual preparation prior to class and group collaboration during a class session. In order for most team-based approaches to be effective, students must arrive to their teams prepared with information and ready to engage with their teammates.

Some disciplines have very specific interpretations of team-based learning that use a highly structured approach with multiple assessments. These include individual quizzes (readiness assessment tests), team quizzes (team readiness assessment tests) and verbal or written appeals for wrong answers. Some approaches use instant grading (using scratch off cards to reveal answers) and simultaneous reporting of answers (using placards for multiple choice or true/false question) that can foster a competitive atmosphere. Assessments are also incorporated for students to grade teammates, measure accountability, or reflect on learning preferences and satisfaction.

The fundamental concept of team-based learning offers flexibility for interpretation. Ideas from the highly structured team-based learning activities can be incorporated into distance learning to provide opportunities for collaborative learning that include informal and formative assessment. In distance learning, team-based learning can be executed in synchronous courses using videoconferencing. The chat feature or breakout rooms can be used for deliberations. In hybrid courses, team interaction can take place during face-to-face class meetings or asynchronously by creating groups in discussion forums.

One feature of team-based learning that encourages a true team approach is when a single grade is awarded to each team as a whole unit. A difficulty with this is that it can penalize students in poor performing groups. An alternative is to use multiple assessments that include a grade for teamwork and grades for individual activities. This can provide a more holistic assessment of learning and avoid the possibility that a poor performing group could adversely impact a student's grade.

Balancing time for team-based learning activities can take experimentation. It should allow adequate opportunities for students to exchange ideas. It should also allow students to reference course material when working on team answers. Team-based learning activities can be structured to reinforce how students can utilize different types of resources to support their learning.

Students may struggle with team based learning. They may have difficulty speaking up in their group. Students may feel like they are self-teaching rather than being beneficiaries of instruction. To help address these types of struggles, instructors should continually circulate through the class while teams are working. If groups are not well balanced in terms of contribution, instructors can reconfigure groups for subsequent activities to promote student participation and engagement.

Team-Based Learning Example 1

This activity could replace a lecture in anatomy & physiology on the nervous system.

For pre-work students read a textbook chapter(s) on the nervous system. Each student takes a 10 question multiple choice quiz. The quiz questions should be complex in a way that requires students to carefully consider possible answers. Students take the quiz online but do not receive a grade (yet.)

Upon arrival in class students work on the same quiz as a team. Each team must use negotiation and peer teaching to agree on a single answer to each question. Students must find a way to negotiate within their team to agree upon one answer. This could be by voting on an answer, assigning students different questions, or another strategy. The online quiz must be configured: a) so that it is timed to be completed in a specified period of time, and b) one team member can submit answers on behalf of the team, and c) the quiz is automatically graded to reveal the correct and incorrect answers to each team.

Next the entire class comes together with the instructor to review the quiz. Any group that got an answer incorrect is given the opportunity to appeal their answer to the instructor and the class. The appeals process stimulates discussion and serves as a review of course material that needs clarification. This appeal does not alter the grade on the quiz; but it helps students work through rationale for the incorrect answer and find a pathway to the correct answer.

After the appeals process, the instructor can conduct a short lecture covering topics that require further review/clarification.

To end the class, each student takes a second 10 question quiz covering material from the chapter. If possible, this quiz should be set up for automatic grading so that students can get immediate feedback. After class, students can see their individual grade on the first quiz.

This approach to team based learning provides multiple opportunities for assessments. Two quizzes provide individual grades in addition to the team quiz grade. By including multiple assessments it decreases the potential that students may be penalized by a poor team performance. Repeated use of quizzes throughout the activity can help students become more comfortable with test taking.

Team-Based Learning Example 2

This activity could replace a pathophysiology or kinesiology lecture. Reviews of movement videos are analyzed throughout to provide visual references for students.

Students read a textbook chapter or watch a recorded presentation on joint movements and common injuries. Prior to class each student completes a 10-question multiple choice quiz that reviews material from the chapter or presentation.

The live class uses video clips and a polling app for an interactive quiz. The video clips should be a few seconds in duration and show complex movements (e.g. downhill skier on a moguls course, farmhand picking vegetables, delivery person loading a box onto a truck) that allow the movements to be shown in a loop. Each video clip is accompanied by 2 to 3 questions with multiple choice answers.

The class watches a video and then moves to small group teams (in breakout rooms) for a 10-minute deliberation to answer each question for that video. Teams must negotiate a single answer to each question. Team answers can be submitted to the LMS for each question to provide a record for grading.

The class comes back together and the instructor presents each question as a poll. All students respond with their team's answers. The poll reveals the answer distribution. Teams have the opportunity to defend or appeal their answer. This will promote review and class discussion, after which the instructor reveals the correct answer.

The class watches another video, and repeats the team deliberations, followed by another poll and appeal discussion. This can be repeated several times to work through different video clips.

Each student's quiz and the team answers to the polling/interactive quiz provide assessments for grading. Students can also complete a self-assessment to reflect on how they used the preparation work (readings or recorded presentation), team deliberation, and class discussions as part of their learning process.

Team-Based Learning Example 3

This activity could replace a lecture in pathophysiology. Instead of an appeals process, peer teaching is used to foster collaboration within the class.

To prepare, students read a textbook chapter.

Before class, students complete a quiz that requires short answers (3 to 5 sentences each.)

When class begins, each team collaborates on a 10 question quiz that references information from the short answer quiz already completed by each student. Students can compare and contrast their short answers and also use other course materials. The team quiz should be set up to use a designated responder for each team and automatic grading.

The class comes back together and team scores are revealed. The lowest performing team is given the first chance to seek clarification for a question. They confer to select the question and ask another team to explain the correct answer. After that explanation, the instructor can request that a second explanation is provided from another team. If needed, the instructor can provide a summary and direct the class to specific resources in class materials.

Next, the second lowest performing team can select a different question and a team to provide an explanation for the correct answer. This process continues until each of the 10 questions has been explained.

All teams should be given the opportunity to explain at least one correct answer. The peer teaching approach used here instead of the traditional appeals process to the instructor gives students a chance to learn through teaching. The ability to use peer teaching relies on the assumption that no team will get all 10 questions wrong.

After the peer-teaching activity concludes, students complete an evaluation of peer teaching by the other teams. This evaluation, the individual short answer quiz, and the team quiz provide multiple assessments for the activity.

Project-Based Learning

Project-based learning is an applied or extended learning experience that results in production of a product. This product should have some application either within the course or to a realistic scenario so that the activity does not feel like busy work. Project-based learning can be individualized or involve group projects. In distance learning, group project-based learning provides multiple opportunities for engagement between instructors and students and for interaction among students.

The process of project-based learning should provide students with the opportunity to explore, apply, and integrate course concepts and material while working towards the goal of producing something. It can be done on a small scale by having students draft a study guide, develop a quiz, or create a handout. Larger projects such as a presentation or research paper can be completed in stages over the length of a course or term to nest smaller learning within the larger project. Regardless of the size of the project, the process should include scaffolding so that students complete it in stages with a timeline and framework to help them stay on track.

Project-based learning can be incorporated into a class at any stage in the curriculum. For introductory or foundational courses it can be used to review material. For advanced courses it can encourage integration of knowledge by requiring students to leverage information from foundational courses. Project-based learning can also serve as a culminating learning experience that requires students to apply and integrate information from across the curriculum. Client education and marketing materials can be especially useful projects as students near completion of a course or program.

The beginning of project-based learning should allow time for students to get organized. For individual projects students will need time to gather resources and identify resource gaps. For group activities, group members will need time to brainstorm and negotiate roles. If topics are not assigned, students should be given time to decide on a topic.

Having students take turns sharing their projects with the class offers several benefits. Students can receive peer feedback. This is especially important in distance learning where there is little opportunity for casual interaction that would typically occur on campus.

Articulating a project requires organization of ideas, which can help students see progress. Presentations allow students to learn from each other. When a project extends or expands course material, it offers an opportunity for advanced learning.

Multiple assessments can be incorporated into project-based learning. For example grades and feedback on a draft of the project, a presentation, and the final product create a holistic assessment and provide insight into how students work with feedback. For individual projects students can complete a self-evaluation or reflection. For group projects students can be asked to provide a self-assessment,, an evaluation of their group's function as a unit, and an assessment of their contribution to the overall group effort.

It is relatively easy to create a small project for a single course. The examples provided here are more complex. They were prepared to show how problem-based learning can integrate material from different areas. When all groups are working on the same complex problem, it can be helpful for the class to see different approaches and different solutions.

Project-Based Learning Example 1

This activity could be used as an interactive session to replace lectures on clinical reasoning, business, and ethics.

This example uses a scenario of a ballet company that is expanding services to help dancers manage routine soreness and discomfort. Students are presented with a scenario for a group project. This example could also be adapted for an individual project.

The ballet company plans to offer personal training 6 days per week in the afternoons by a full-time employee. A system is needed to organize appointments, maintain records, conduct assessments, and track progress. Information about the training sessions may need to be shared with physical therapists who are also employees of the ballet company. Record keeping should include a summary of each dancer's symptoms, description of assessments performed, results of the assessments, and a description of the training activities.

Dancers in the company have different needs. One of the apprentice dancers is a 17-year old male with persistent groin pain. A 15-year old female apprentice has chronic low back discomfort and suffers from headaches. A 34-year old principal dancer has a history of tibial stress fracture, dancer's fracture, and ankle sprain.

Students are asked to prepare a summary of the proposed program, list of required resources and supplies, and an appointment schedule that includes time for training sessions and conducting record keeping activities.

After each group has completed their summary, all groups take turns reporting to the class. The instructor and other students can seek clarifications and make suggestions. Each group receives a grade for their summary and presentation. Students can self-assess their own contribution.

Problem-Based Learning Example 2

This activity could replace lectures on sports injuries in pathophysiology class as well as lectures on business and ethics. As presented, students could have several synchronous meetings to work through different aspects of the scenario.

This activity uses a scenario of a minor league professional baseball team that is expanding its medical staff to hire a full-time strength and conditioning specialist. Students are tasked with doing research to prepare a job description.

> This role of the strength and conditioning specialist will involve collaboration with team physicians, athletic trainers, strength and conditioning coaches, and physical therapists during training and regular baseball season. Attendance at a daily medical team meeting is required. Travel with the team to away games is required. All supplies needed for training will be provided by the team.

> The team roster changes every year. Players on the current team roster are males between the ages of 18 and 32. For 20 percent of the current team, English is a second language. The team provides interpreters during practice and games. Players on the current team and in years past have similar problems including: rotator cuff injuries, arm soreness or tendinitis in the hand, elbow, or shoulder, and hamstring strains. All medical treatments are scheduled on an as-needed basis for players before team practice sessions and prior to games on game day.

For this activity students are asked to identify types of problems and injuries the strength and conditioning specialist is likely to encounter, summarize techniques and tools that could be used to treat the players, and provide references to support evidence for different approaches. Next groups are asked to propose individual or group session schedules for players depending upon whether they are at risk for an injury, coping with an injury, or recovering.

After each group has completed their investigation, each group will prepare a job description for the strength and conditioning specialist. It should include required knowledge and skills as well as scheduling, salary, and benefit information.

Groups take turns reporting their job descriptions to the class and providing rationale based upon their investigation. After all groups have presented, the class can compare and contrast the job descriptions, information gathered, and sources used for information. Each group receives a grade for their job description. Students can self-assess their own contribution.

Problem-Based Learning Example 3

This activity could replace lectures in pathophysiology, kinesiology, business, and ethics classes. As a complex problem, portions can be broken down to have students spend time collaborating to research different employee needs, evidence for treatment options, considerations for employee wellness program designs, and proposal formats.

Students are presented with a scenario for an employee wellness program. This activity requires students to develop a research-informed proposal for a fitness program that is being developed as part of the program.

> Management of a large manufacturing company is proposing a comprehensive employee wellness program. Employees that work in the manufacturing facility are at risk for repetitive stress injuries from work-related movements. Employees who work in administrative roles within the company are primarily desk workers who sit most of the workday.

> The overarching goals of the wellness program are health promotion and stress management. The company is renovating space for a wellness center. It will include a group activity room, a private office space, and restroom facilities. The company is seeking competitive proposals for a contractor to work part-time to run a fitness program for employees in the private office space.

Students are asked to prepare a proposal for a 6 month pilot test for a corporate fitness program. The proposal should provide a description of types of sessions that can be scheduled by employees on breaks during the workday. The proposal should take into account any specific knowledge and skills needed, and assessments that will be used, to meet the needs of employees who work in different roles within the company. Evidence-based material should be referenced to support ideas. The proposal should include a basic budget with start-up costs (for equipment and supplies), cleaning, maintenance, and salaries. The schedule should provide information about appointment scheduling and detail time needed for cleaning and recordkeeping in between sessions.

The instructor or facilitator can help guide the students to learn about repetitive stress injuries and workplace wellness in manufacturing. For the learning activity, a proposal template can be provided or groups can be required to find a resource to create their own proposal format.

Each group should prepare a brief presentation summarizing their proposal—as if they were to present to company management. Groups can present their proposals to the class.

In addition to a grade for the final proposal each student in the class can grade presentations by other groups, give feedback to members of their own group, and do a self-assessment on their contribution. These grades can be averaged to contribute to the overall grade.

Problem-Based Learning

Problem-based learning is a teaching approach that draws upon realistic, complex scenarios that take students through a facilitated process to apply course concepts and arrive at a solution. While problem-based learning can be individualized, it can also involve small groups collaborating to work through complex problems. The goal of the activity can be either to propose a solution, or to choose a solution from options provided.

The discussion and use of resources in problem-based learning activities provides the chance for students to explore and apply course material and concepts. While lecture-based teaching presents information first then follows with assessment later, problem-based learning works the other way around. Students are presented with a problem. As they research background information and explore possible solutions, more information is revealed that could influence suggested solutions.

Different interpretations of problem-based learning are used in academic disciplines including medicine, engineering, and business. Some of the approaches are highly structured and included semester-long group work, case scenarios, or dedicated faculty serving as facilitator/tutor. Various adaptations and interpretations of problem-based learning all have one thing in common: collective thinking about a solution. Ideas from the more structured and formal approaches to problem-based learning can be used to create engaging distance learning sessions. Problem-based learning works well using a multi-stage process that employs a framework to provide opportunities for exploration.

Fundamental components of problem-based learning are defining the problem, gathering information, seeking out additional resources to explore ideas, collaborating to think through solutions, negotiating within their group, defending their answers, and arriving at a conclusion as a group. An overarching goal of problem-based learning is for students to recognize how to use critical thinking skills in combination with self-directed learning in pursuit of a solution. The group aspect of problem-based learning presents opportunities for peer teaching and mutual accountability.

Sources of material for problem-based learning should be intriguing and relevant to engage students. Timely topics or critical issues can promote information literacy as students work on identifying the right types of resources to answer questions. Complexity of the problem is essential so students are required to seek out information and engage in deliberation within their group.

Facilitation in the problem-based learning activity by the instructor helps guide students through the process. For a small class the instructor can facilitate multiple groups. For larger classes multiple facilitators will be needed or the sessions scheduled at different times to allow the instructor to spend time facilitating each group. When different facilitators will participate in the activity, training and orientation is needed ahead of time to ensure consistency in the facilitation.

Problem-based learning can be designed for an entire 2 to 3 hour class or as a portion of a class meeting. Depending upon the length of time used for the small group discussions, multiple scenarios could be covered in a single 3 hour class. If the entire session cannot be accommodated in a single synchronous meeting, a combination of asynchronous activities (e.g. discussion forums, collaborative documents, homework) can be used for small group work.

Problem-Based Learning Example 1

This activity could replace a lecture in pathophysiology. It could also be used as an introduction to a practicum. The scenario used should have multiple possible answers. This activity focuses on the problem solving process, use of resource material, and rationale for their answer.

To begin class, a scenario is presented for a client with persistent, unexplained back pain.

Working in small groups, students summarize what they know about potential risk factors for back pain. Each group is asked to identify three questions that would help them learn more. The questions are recorded and a reporter assigned from within the group.

The class reconvenes and each group takes turns sharing their three questions. Next the instructor provides more information about the client to reveal more about the scenario (e.g. there is no history of back injury, the pain has been intermittent for over 4 months, results from active and passive range of motion tests.)

The small groups confer to revisit the scenario again with the new information. They can consider whether the questions supplied by other groups suggests something they might have overlooked. They can mark resources from course materials or elsewhere to guide a decision.

The class reconvenes and the instructor presents a multiple choice question with potential next steps for the client scenario. There should be no single correct answer, but different options with potential risks and benefits. An example of a question for which the students deliberate an answer would be the following:

Under which of the following circumstances could a training session for the client proceed:

- Simultaneous hip and trunk flexion cause acute pain in the posterior thigh.

- No back pain is present when seated in a chair, but acute pain occurs when rising to a standing position.

- The pain started after the client underwent bariatric surgery 6 months ago.

- The client is taking medication and participating in psychotherapy for depression.

Small groups discuss possible answers for 10 minutes and agree on their answer.

The class reconvenes and all groups submit their answer. This can be done by having a designated reporter from each group state their response using a roll call. The instructor calls on groups with similar answers to provide rationale for their answer to the class and share resources used.

Once all groups have answered, the instructor can summarize the potential risks and benefits of each answer.

For scenarios that do not have a single correct answer, a grading rubric can be used to evaluate each group on the rationale provided to support their answer choice. Students can assess their own performance by summarizing their major contribution to the group effort and indicating what percentage their individual effort represents of the total effort by their group.

Problem-Based Learning Example 2

This activity could replace a lecture in anatomy & physiology or pathophysiology. This example begins as an in-class activity, includes homework assignments, and continues over several class sessions.

Prior to the first class students watch a recorded presentation that introduces DENTS, a step-wise problem-solving model: Define, Explore, Narrow the possibilities, and Test a hypothesis, to find a Solution

(DENTS.) A handout that accompanies the presentation provides a one-page worksheet that will be completed in class.

Students are assigned to small groups to evaluate a statement as true or false. The whole class should work on the same statement during a session. Each group should submit a completed DENTS worksheet at the conclusion of the activity.

The first class begins with presentation of a statement. The statement can be a misconception, myth, or attempt to link a cause and effect to a heath outcome. The statements should be somewhat broad in order to require students to choose a specific aspect of the statement to investigate. Example: anxiety increases pain.

Students begin by working in small groups for 15 to 20 minutes to *define* and *explore* the statement. Each group should assign a recorder to complete the DENTS worksheet on behalf of the group. Students next look for reference material related to the statement. Groups can use a folder or discussion forum in the LMS to share ideas.

In the second class small groups spend 20 to 30 minutes in discussion. Each group uses information from their homework to help the group *narrow* their exploration to a specific area related to the statement that could be supported (or refuted) by research. At the conclusion of the group discussion period, a reporter from each group shares with the class the specific area the group will investigate and their hypothesis. Examples:

- Sympathetic nervous system arousal facilitates transmission of pain signals.

- Individuals with anxiety disorders experience higher levels of pain during dental appointments.

- Interventions to reduce anxiety decreased reported pain for patients undergoing cancer treatment.

Homework to prepare for the third class is for group members to *test their hypothesis* by finding evidence to support or refute their hypothesis. Depending upon the level of the class, this could include sections of course materials, expert recommendations from reputable sources, first-person reports, suggestions from professional or patient advocacy groups, and/or peer-reviewed research articles. The exploration should lead to a *solution* to support whether the original statement was true or false.

In the third class small groups spend 20 to 30 minutes completing their DENTS worksheet including 3-5 references that they used to evaluate their hypothesis. Based upon their findings the group must come to a conclusion on whether the original statement was true or false.

The fourth class begins with the instructor reading the statement. All groups report whether they concluded that the statement was true or false. This can be done with a representative from each group responding to a roll call.

Next there is a class discussion/debate. A reporter from each group gives a 2 to 3 minute summary of the group's narrowing, hypothesis test, and results. Reports from groups should be clustered by the group's answer.

After all groups have reported, each provides an answer to the true/false statement that includes a 3-5 sentence rationale.

Multiple assessments can be used for this activity. Each group's DENTS worksheet can be assessed. Students can self-assess their participation and contribution to their group. Students can also grade other group contributions to the final discussion/debate.

Problem-Based Learning Example 3

This activity could replace a lecture in an ethics course.

Class begins with a presentation of an ethical scenario (e.g. laptop is stolen that contains client records, sexual harassment accusation by a colleague, discrimination against potential client, etc.) This can be provided to students as a one page summary that initially only contains very basic information about the problem.

Students work in small groups for 15 to 20 minutes to prepare a structured response to: a) summarize their understanding of the situation, b) identify the ethical problem presented, and c) propose a next step to work towards a solution.

The class comes together and the instructor reveals more information about the scenario (e.g. the client records included credit card numbers, the accusation is against a manager, the client believes the discrimination was racial bias.) Students are given a few minutes to ask questions or request clarifications.

The small groups reconvene and review their structured response and consider the newly acquired information. They spend 15 to 20 minutes gathering resource material that could help inform a solution.

The class comes together and the instructor presents a multiple choice question with potential next steps to work toward a solution for the scenario. There is one correct answer, but it should not be obvious. Other answer options should be worded to encourage debate.

Small groups have 10 minutes to debate their answer.

The class reconvenes and all groups submit their answer. This can be done by having a designated reporter from each draw the letter corresponding to their answer on a card. All reporters simultaneously reveal their answers. The instructor calls on groups with similar answers to provide rationale for their answer to the class. This should include discussion of resource material that was used to arrive at the answer.

After the discussion, the instructor reveals the correct answer. This should be followed by a brief lecture that provides an explanation, rationale, and a recommended list of resources that the groups could have used.

A rubric can be used to grade each group on their structured response and quality of resource materials referenced. Students can self-assess their contribution to the group.

Peer Teaching

Peer teaching is a learning strategy designed to have students learning from and with each other in a designated activity. It can be used to create interactive instructional sessions for students to engage with each other. Peer teaching provides a unique type of support. It can be helpful to have someone different provide a definition, explain a concept, or lead a review. When students relate to each other it can provide social and emotional support.

For complicated course material, incorporating peer teaching can provide students in a large class with some individualized instruction. Students can reinforce their own knowledge by teaching. Introducing peer teaching to a course helps students migrate away from dependence on a course instructor.

There are different approaches for peer teaching. A unidirectional approach is to have advanced students serve as surrogate teachers to tutor struggling students. A multidirectional approach uses cooperative and reciprocal peer teaching that is done with students taking turns as teachers and learners for different sessions or topics.

In distance learning, small group peer teaching can be used to provide multiple opportunities for engagement. Students in small groups can engage with each other. Then the small groups can report back to the class on strategies used or information learned.

There are multiple possibilities for assessments for peer teaching. The peer teachers can produce a learning aid. Students can evaluate their peer teacher. When students serve in the role as peer teachers, they can complete a self-reflection.

Peer Teaching Example 1

This activity could be used as a review for any course. It can replace an instructor review session or an open session where students would simply ask questions of the instructor.

This is a variation of Just in Time instruction. It uses an informal assessment to identify topics that students know well and material that needs review or revisiting. To prepare, the instructor creates a list of topics that will be covered on an end of unit exam. The list can be formatted as an ungraded quiz or an online survey. Students are asked to review the list and identify two topics they know well enough to teach and two topics for which they need clarification or help. Students should complete the survey 24-48 hours before class.

The instructor reviews the responses to identify: a) topics that a majority of students need reviewed, b) topics that can be used to form small groups for review. From the lists, the instructor can form small groups for peer teaching. Each group will contain one or two students who know a topic well (assigned as peer teachers) and students who need clarification or help on that topic. Time permitting, two peer teaching sessions can be held during class, each with different small groups and different peer teachers.

At the beginning of class the instructor spends 15 to 20 minutes reviewing topics that required clarification from the majority of the class. This can include suggestions for what course materials or supplemental resources students can revisit while studying.

After the small group, the class can come together for a 15-minute debriefing. One student from each group can be asked to share something from the peer teaching in their group. It can be new insights, information that was helpful, or material that they will need to spend more time studying. This can be followed by debriefing and closing remarks from the instructor to conclude the class session.

Time permitting, a second round of peer teaching can be held with different groups and topics following the same format.

Every student may not be perfectly matched to topics; they may be assigned to a small group with a topic they did not choose. But all students will likely benefit from a review session that is interactive. All topics will not necessarily be covered. But this format allows for more information to be covered in a targeted way. It also helps the instructor identify material that the majority of students feel requires clarification.

Students can complete a self-reflection for an assessment. They can describe what they learned in their group and outline a plan to study concepts they need to review.

Peer Teaching Example 2

This activity could replace a lecture in anatomy & physiology, pathophysiology, or kinesiology.

This format is highly interactive. It requires pre-class preparation and organization during the session to keep students on task and on time. A multiple topic, team-based approach used for peer teaching works well for topics that are related to each other or have some overlap. Complex topics can provide the opportunity for students to apply and integrate information. Examples:

- Chemotherapy-associated peripheral neuropathy and diabetic neuropathy

- Osteoarthritis and rheumatoid arthritis

- Multiple sclerosis and dystonia

- Chronic fatigue syndrome and fibromyalgia

BEYOND LECTURES

This format is highly interactive. It requires pre-class preparation and organization during the session to keep students on task and on time.

To prepare for class students are assigned to one of two topics (Topic A or Topic B.) Within each topic, students are assigned to small groups forming teaching teams to serve as peer teachers. Each peer teaching team prepares a 10-15 minute teaching session for their topic. This should include a handout, slides, or other resource used as teaching material. All students should play a role in the peer teaching session either in preparation of material, presenting, or answering questions.

To begin class, peer teaching teams from Topic A are paired with teams from Topic B. Groups move to a 20 minute breakout session to teach Topic A.

The whole class comes together for a summary of Topic A. Peer teaching groups can each take a turn sharing key points or information.

Groups move to a second 20 minute breakout session to where teams from Topic B teach to the teams from Topic A.

The whole class again comes together for a summary of Topic B. Again peer teaching groups can each take a turn sharing key points.

Next the instructor uses a poll to have the class take a brief interactive quiz on both topics. If topics have some overlap, the quiz can compare and contrast the topics. For each question after all students have answered, the instructor can review the correct answer for the class.

This activity provides multiple opportunities for assessments. The teaching materials supplied by each peer teaching team can be graded. Students can complete a self-assessment of their contribution to the peer teaching activity. Students can evaluate their team members. Students can also evaluate effectiveness of the team that taught the other topic.

Peer Teaching Example 3

This activity uses a designated reader approach. Each student in the small group can take a turn serving as the designated reader and peer teacher for a session.

All students are assigned to small groups for the duration of the course. During each unit in the course, one session on peer teaching can be conducted giving each student a chance to be the peer teacher. The peer teacher serves as the designated reader for a textbook chapter or other substantial reading assignment.

To prepare for the session the peer teacher prepares a one-page reference guide or short slide presentation for their small group. This should contain important terms, bullet points on material covered in the reading, and perhaps drawings or illustrations. The reference guide should be brief but comprehensive. It can be submitted as an assignment prior to class.

To begin class, the instructor outlines the topics that each designated reader intends to cover. All students should be given access to reference guides created by the designated readers for the session.

Each designated reader leads a 15 to 20 minute tutorial on the reading using their reference guide or slide presentation to provide a summary of the reading. This should include time for questions and answers about material. Any questions that the designated reader cannot answer should be written down to share with the course instructor.

The class reconvenes and the designated peer teacher for each group can provide a short summary of material covered in their group.

Next, all students take a short online quiz in the LMS on the material from the assigned reading. If possible the quiz should be formatted for automatic grading so the instructor can review the grades immediately. Class can conclude with the instructor reviewing answers to the quiz.

This activity provides multiple assessment opportunities. A grading rubric can be used to evaluate the discussion guide prepared by the designated reader. Each student's quiz score would serve as an assessment. All students can be asked to evaluate the designated reader for their group.

Simulation

Simulation is an instructional method that requires participants to navigate a fictional situation that approximates a real-world scenario. The context and setting for a simulation generally has defined parameters. Students can work individually or in groups to solve problems or to practice skills. In some areas of education, simulation has evolved into elaborate sessions that take place in staged environments with actors hired to play roles in the activity (e.g. standard patients used in healthcare simulations.) Sometimes simulation is structured to involve interaction among students from different disciplines or professions (interprofessional education.) The overall approach is the same: role play in a real-world scenario.

On a fundamental level, simulation engages students in the psychomotor domain of learning by providing space to practice skills and making decisions while learning. Participation in simulation creates a safe space for learning through action and experimentation. Activities that require analysis, choices, and rationale behind choices can help students develop critical thinking skills. Simulation is immersive.

Creative teaching using simulation can require students to apply and integrate concepts from anatomy & physiology, pathophysiology, and kinesiology. One important aspect of simulation is defining the student's role so that it provides an optimal learning experience in a way that is relevant to the course. When role play is used for simulation students should not assume the role of a different healthcare provider or other professional for purposes of the activity. While that might be interesting, it can be confusing for students who are working to develop their own professional identity.

The examples provided here could be adapted for use in an online platform (e.g. VirBELA, Mursion, zSpace, or Open Simulator) to have students role play using avatars. If a platform outside of the typical synchronous meeting method is used, all participants should have the opportunity to practice and ensure that they are able to meet technical requirements prior to the class meeting for the simulation session.

For small classes breakout sessions would not be necessary if the activity can be structured to accommodate participation by the entire class. For large classes, the simulations can use small groups. Members of the class can take turns as participants in the simulation or as observers. Alternatively the simulations can be scheduled at different times.

A simulation session should be designed based upon specific learning objectives. The session should provide an overview for students that reviews the objectives and orients them to the space where the simulation will take place. It is customary to hold a debriefing immediately after a simulation to give students a chance to reflect on their participation and get feedback from the instructor. After all students have participated in the simulation, the instructor can lead a debriefing for the whole class.

Assessments should be used to ensure that students actively participate in the simulation and that they take it seriously. For an informal assessment, students can grade themselves on a rubric. Instructors can use a rubric to assess student performance in the simulation and identify areas where there is room for students to grow.

Simulation Example 1

This activity could replace a lecture in pathophysiology or practicum.

In a professional setting health history forms are often lengthy and time to interview clients is short. Simulation using role play can help students practice conducting client interviews to hone their skills. The objective of this simulation is for students to learn how to identify important information that might be relevant to exercise program design and tailor interview questions to maximize information that can be gleaned in a short amount of time.

The instructor prepares background information for a series of case scenarios. Each scenario should be realistic in nature. The simulation format provides a good opportunity to role play questions on common conditions like hypertension, diabetes, and back pain. There should be information embedded in the scenario to ensure that the activity provides a learning experience for the class.

With the instructor playing the role of the client in the scenario, a student is assigned to conduct a timed interview to gather information needed to plan a single introductory exercise session. Other students observe. In a small class this activity can be used in different classes allowing all students to take a turn as an interviewer in the simulation. Depending on whether the students are novices or more experienced, the instructor can structure responses to make the simulation straight forward or more complex.

After the simulated interview concludes, polling can be used for review and discussion. A few (2 or 3) multiple choice or true/false questions can cover program design or precautions for the condition that was used in the role play. The questions should be structured so that there is no single obvious correct answer, but different possibilities to invite debate. Students can be asked to provide rationale for their answers to promote discussion in the class.

This can be followed by an instructor-facilitated debriefing focused on the interview structure used by the student. Students who participate in the role play can complete a self-assessment of their performance and identify areas for growth. A grading rubric can be used to assess each student's performance.

Simulation Example 2

This activity could be used in place of a lecture in pathophysiology or practicum.

Reviewing scenarios and practicing interviews provides an opportunity for students to gather information and get insight from other students. This simulation uses a crowd-sourced approach to selecting and practicing interview questions. Students get an opportunity for an in depth review of the signs, symptoms, or diagnosed disorder presented in the scenario in addition to the role play simulation.

A brief prerecorded video is prepared using a fictional client narrative. This describes a client's experience with signs, symptoms, or a diagnosed disorder. Complex conditions (e.g. chronic fatigue syndrome, multiple sclerosis, fibromyalgia, complex regional pain syndrome) work well in this activity. The instructor can choose a published narrative or write a narrative for the activity. The instructor could ask a friend or colleague to record the narrative to help delineate the role of the client in the simulation.

The class views the video and students are required to take notes on the scenario. Then the class divides into small groups.

Each small group works for 15 minutes to identify relevant information from the narrative and prepare a list of 5 to 7 questions to include in the interview. These questions should seek clarifications or more information related to the presentation that could help guide decisions for an exercise program. Each group appoints one student to be the interviewer and another to be the designated responder.

The class comes back together and the groups work in sequence. The appointed students from one group role play one interview question. The interviewer seeks an answer from the designated responder in their group. The class observes the interaction. The next group must select a different interview question from their list. The appointed students from that group role play that interview and response. This continues until all groups have contributed a question and answer. Each group must listen carefully to the other groups because they will need to select a question from their list that does not duplicate information already asked by another group.

After each group has asked a question, the class views the prerecorded scenario a second time.

Next another round of simulated interviews is conducted with the interviewer and the designated responder from each group. The interview question from each group should not duplicate information already revealed by previous questions.

After each group has asked a question, the class can view the prerecorded scenario one more time.

The instructor then leads the class in a debriefing. This can include a summary of what the questions and answers revealed about the scenario. It should include general feedback to all groups about the quality and structure of their questions.

This activity could be assessed by grading the list of questions created by each group. Students can complete evaluations of their own group and reflect on their own contributions.

Simulation Example 3

This activity could be used as a follow up to a lecture in pathophysiology or practicum to help students learn about a specific medical condition.

This activity uses case scenarios and role play to help students refine interview questions. The overarching goal is to help students recognize how open ended questions can provide greater insight than binary (Yes/No) questions or checklists. The activity uses improvised interviews which requires the participants in the simulation to think on their feet.

To prepare for the session, the instructor selects a published case scenario or writes a case scenario about a specific medical condition. Common or complex conditions work well in this activity (e.g. hypertension, joint pain, repetitive use injuries, Parkinson disease.) The medical condition should be kept a secret from the class.

In a small class, this simulation can be used with the whole class. In a larger class, students can work in small groups. Two students are selected to play the role of interviewer and client. The instructor emails the case scenario to the student playing the role of client. Only this student receives the scenario.

Next the student playing the role of interviewer conducts a 5-minute, timed interview asking the client questions for which there can only be "yes" or "no" answers. If the interviewer asks any open ended questions, the client is not allowed to respond. The student playing the role of the client should have access to course materials about the medical condition so they can provide accurate answers.

Students who are observing the role play are instructed to take notes. Once the interview time is ended, the observers are required to write three open-ended questions that could take the place of yes/no questions that were asked by the interviewer.

The student interviewer shares a short summary of what they learned from their questions. Next the observer students can take turns asking open ended questions from their list. The student playing the role of the client supplies answers to the open ended questions.

After several more questions have been answered, the student playing the interviewer summarizes what they learned about the client.

The student who played the role of the client then shares the medical condition with the whole class. This can be followed by the instructor summarizing key information that should be gleaned from an interview. The class should then discuss differences in the quality of information from yes/no and open ended questions.

The students involved in the role play as interviewer and client can be graded on participation using a rubric. The list of questions from the observers can be used as another assessment.

Observational Learning

Observational learning is a social learning process. It naturally occurs during growth and development as children watch and mimic others to learn what behaviors are acceptable in different contexts. In social psychology observational learning is described as having four elements: attention, retention, reproduction, and motivation. These elements outline the process involved in adopting a behavior or to successfully execute behavior change. A person recognizes a behavior, remembers it, attempts the behavior, and then is motivated to repeat the behavior. Although this may seem tangential, it describes how watching something can lead to a learning experience which can then influence performance.

While observational learning has a specific definition used in social psychology, the general concept that a student can learn by watching offers an instructional strategy that can be used in any discipline. Observation can be used to foster critical thinking skills with activities that require students to extract, analyze, and evaluate something. Many topics in exercise science, kinesiology, fitness, and personal training are well suited to observational learning.

Observation Example 1

Body mechanics and ergonomics are associated with repetitive use injuries and increased risk of musculoskeletal injuries. This activity can replace a lecture in pathophysiology or kinesiology. Students can model postures and movements for the class to observe and analyze.

To prepare for class, each student is assigned an occupation or activity that is associated with risk of musculoskeletal disorder. Students research and prepare a summary of postures and movements associated with that occupation/activity and ergonomic aids that workers in the occupation might use. This assignment should be submitted prior to class.

When class convenes, students take turns on webcam demonstrating posture or movements associated with their assigned occupation/activity. The observers review the posture or movements to identify what might be associated with increased risk of musculoskeletal injury.

- Seated desk work is associated with low back pain. Proper chair position and taking frequent breaks can reduce risk of chronic pain.

- Playing piano can contribute to repetitive stress injury in the wrists. Pianists can work on positioning of the forearms and alignment of the wrists.

- Delivery workers are required to do a lot of lifting and carrying. Heavy objects increase risk of back pain. Back belts may be used for support.

After demonstration, the class can come back together to compare and contrast their observations. For a follow up assignment students can be required to locate information on the prevalence of different types of work (or activity) related musculoskeletal injuries.

The summaries prepared by the students and the information resources can be used as assessments for this activity.

Observation Example 2

This activity incorporates a flipped classroom with a student assignment into an active learning session for professionalism or practicum.

Visiting workplaces can help students gain insight into professional practice. It can give them a big picture view of the role a health club, fitness center, or studio plays in service to the community.

In this example a virtual field trip is scheduled for the class by inviting a fitness director, personal trainer, or other professional to give students a video tour of their workplace. The guest is asked to record a 15 minute video walk through of their health club, fitness center, or studio that includes an overview of the characteristics of clients seen in the practice.

To prepare for the class, students are asked to gather data about the community in which the practice is based. This can include demographics, predominant cultural groups, major employers, and other information that can give insights into potential clients and their health needs. This summary should be submitted as an assignment prior to the start of the session.

The class session begins by viewing the video for the virtual field trip. As students watch, they look for information that can give insights into how the health club, fitness center, or studio serves needs of clients in the community. Art and décor might reflect predominant cultural groups, discount programs may be offered to major employers, or the office may be designed to be accessible for a community with a lot of older adults.

At the conclusion of the video, the instructor leads a facilitated discussion for students to share their observations.

Each student's summary of the community can be used for an assessment. Additionally students can be asked to summarize three things they learned on the virtual field trip about connections between the facility and the community.

Observation Example 3

This activity could be used in an ethics or professionalism class to help students weigh options to address problems. Negotiation role play is used to introduce the scenarios for students to observe.

Role play that presents ethical dilemmas can be used to help students develop critical thinking strategies and communication skills. This example involves observation of a role play activity with negotiation between a client and a trainer. Each person wants or needs something.

The instructor prepares two short summaries of a client problem that presents an ethical dilemma: one from the client's perspective and the other from the trainer's perspective. The summaries can be a brief narrative or bullet points that provide enough information for students to do a role play. Each summary describes the scenario from the perspective of the role. Some examples of topics include:

- A client refuses to put their age on a health history form. Without a completed health history form, the trainer is uncertain whether to proceed with session.

- A client asks for nutrition or dietary counseling and is willing to pay extra for the session. The trainer needs the money but knows this is outside of scope of practice.

- A client asks the personal trainer to massage their neck and shoulders at the end of the session. The trainer thinks this is okay but is unsure if this is within scope of practice.

Two student volunteers are asked to role play the scenario. They are each given a summary to study and use as a reference. Neither participant is permitted to see the other's summary. The students role play for 2 to 3 minutes live via webcam. Each is instructed to try to negotiate for what they want (or need) out of the conversation. Other students observe the role play and take notes.

After conclusion of the scenario the observers are asked to describe the ethical dilemma they observed. Then the participants in the role play provide context that was included in the summary each received. The observers then give feedback to the practitioner about negotiation strategies that were effective and offer ideas on other ways to address the dilemma.

The instructor can finish the session with a debriefing and a reminder of common ethical challenges that may arise in professional practice.

A follow up to the activity can be used for an assessment by asking all students to summarize the dilemma and outline resources that would help them bolster the trainer's position to resolve the issue and retain the client.

Kinesthetic Instruction

Kinesthetic instruction uses movement and motion. It can be used to guide students to make connections with course material. Demonstrating and cuing exercises is an essential part of exercise science and personal training education, but kinesthetic instruction can also be used to reinforce foundational concepts. Kinesthetic instruction can be used to help students recall, use, and apply concepts from anatomy, physiology, and kinesiology. Incorporating kinesthetic learning activities provides students with a multisensory experience to help them embody information. Activities used in face-to-face classrooms can be easily adapted to synchronous distance learning. For example, students can palpate muscle origins and insertions or trace the direction of muscle fibers with a piece of yarn. Students perform joint movements with and without resistance to recognize differences between muscle coactivation and motor unit recruitment. Simultaneous demonstration of multi joint movements can help students recognize how bodies move differently.

Kinesthetic instruction requires that students have adequate space to move. They should be dressed in clothing and footwear that accommodates movement. To ensure that students are participating and staying on task, the class and instructor should use webcams for activities. The participatory nature of kinesthetic instruction can make a class session fun. Making connections between kinesthetic activities and movement science or health is essential to promote critical thinking. To get students to take a kinesthetic class seriously, assessments should be incorporated.

Kinesthetic Instruction Example 1

Prior to class students review muscular anatomy and complete an assignment to create a study resource. The resource should be designed to allow them to look up information quickly. It can be a slide deck, spreadsheet, table in a document, or set of flash cards. The resource will be used during a quiz in the synchronous class session.

The instructor creates a 10 question quiz on muscles and movements. An answer sheet for the quiz can be posted in the LMS for students to download. Using the shoulder as an example, possible quiz questions might include:

- What movement eccentrically contracts serratus anterior?

- What action of the shoulder does not involve pectoralis major?

- What movement concentrically contracts a muscle that works across two joints?

The quiz questions can be shown on a slide and read aloud. Students are given time to demonstrate a movement on webcam then fill out their answer sheet with the movement they performed and connect that movement to an everyday activity. At the end of the quiz, all students upload their answer sheets to the LMS for grading.

Assessments for this activity can include the study resource the students developed and the grade on the quiz.

Kinesthetic Instruction Example 2

A lecture on the cardiovascular system could be enhanced with kinesthetic instruction to help students understand changes that occur in the circulatory and respiratory systems upon exertion. Simple cardiorespiratory fitness testing is used to gather data for the activity.

Prior to class, students read a textbook chapter or material on cardiovascular and respiratory anatomy & physiology. Students are asked to dress in clothing and footwear that accommodates movement and ensure that there is ample space in view of the webcam to allow them to participate. A worksheet can be prepared for students to record information during the activity. NOTE: students who have medical conditions that require precautions during exercise or exertion should observe this activity but not participate.

To begin class, students are shown how to take their radial pulse. Each student records their heart rate while sitting quietly. They are also asked to record their rate of perceived exertion on the traditional Borg scale from 6 (not exerting at all) to 20 (working very, very hard.)

Students are instructed to stand facing their webcam. The first activity is marching in place for 5 minutes. The instructor times the activity and encourages the students to keep marching until time is up. At the conclusion of 5 minutes, students record their rate of perceived exertion and their radial pulse.

The next activity is jogging in place for 5 minutes. Students that struggle to jog can be encouraged to alternate jogging with marching or walking. The instructor times the activity and encourages students to keep moving until time is up. At the conclusion of 5 minutes, students record their rate of perceived exertion and their radial pulse.

Students now have data to analyze for an assignment. The instructor can show the class how to make a table to compare their heart rate and rate of perceived exertion at rest, while marching, and while jogging. After the data are entered into the table, students can add a zero to each rate of perceived exertion number to compare that to their heart rate. The completed data sheets can be uploaded to the LMS to be used as an assessment.

This activity can be followed by the instructor giving a short presentation on cardiorespiratory response to exercise and exertion.

Kinesthetic Instruction Example 3

A lecture in kinesiology on isotonic and isometric muscle contractions can be enhanced by having students perform movements.

To prepare for class students are asked to dress in clothing and footwear that accommodates movement. The instructor should prepare an answer sheet for students to write down answers during the activity.

To begin class, the instructor reviews characteristics of isotonic and isometric muscle contraction. Definitions and descriptions can be placed on a slide or handout for students to view.

Students are asked to stand or sit in view of their webcam. Students should ensure that there is ample space in view of the webcam to allow them to move freely. The instructor should be able to see the gallery of students.

The instructor calls out the name of a movement and the students are required to do two things: demonstrate an everyday activity that incorporates the movement and connect the movement to an exercise. Six to eight different types of movements can be used for a 20 to 30 minute session.

Examples might include:

- Isotonic shoulder flexion could be demonstrated by sweeping the floor and connected to dumbbell rows.

- Isometric hip flexion could be demonstrated by driving a car and connected to wall sits.

- Isotonic knee extension could be demonstrated by walking up stairs and connected to squats.

After students demonstrate the movement they can write down the activity and the connected exercise on their answer sheets. The answer sheets can be uploaded to the LMS for an assessment.

Next the class reviews the activity. Students can take turns demonstrating the movements and everyday activities they chose to compare and contrast their answers.

The instructor can end the session with a debriefing to encourage students to use movements when they are studying.

Demonstrating Exercise and Practice Teaching

During live, face-to-face laboratory and practicum classes students can easily take turns demonstrating assessments and teaching exercises. Exercise equipment is maintained, assessment tools are calibrated, and facilities have adequate space for learning activities. During face-to-face classes instructors can give feedback to students as they work or immediately after the instructional activity. Some aspects of laboratory and practicum classes in exercise science and personal training can be challenging to execute in distance learning. However, the emergence of virtual teaching by personal trainers and fitness instructors presents an opportunity to reimagine laboratory and practicum activities for online delivery.

When courses need to include performance of assessments or teaching exercises, instructional activities can be adapted. Field tests can be substituted for assessments performed on calibrated equipment. Fitness equipment designed for home use (e.g. handheld weights, resistance bands, and balls) or bodyweight exercises can be substituted for exercises performed on professional grade exercise equipment in a gym or laboratory. Students may need to reconfigure their learning space to allow adequate movement or modify movements to fit available space. Discussing these types of modifications as part of the course can help students learn about tele-healthcare.

Students could prepare short instructional videos demonstrating exercises. The instructor could grade the videos on each student's performance. If students were assigned different exercises to demonstrate, a video repository could be created for the class. A follow up assignment might ask students to select a series of videos to create home-exercise programs for different client scenarios. During a live class, students could work in small groups to compare and contrast their program designs.

One major objection to online teaching of exercises or assessments is liability. This is usually cited as the potential for a student to cause injury if an instructor is not positioned to give feedback to students. It is inadvisable to attempt to teach potentially dangerous techniques without adequate supervision and safeguards in place. Regardless of whether a class is taught in a face-to-face setting or online, students should receive thorough guidance in how to execute and teach exercises. All students should be instructed to speak up if anything causes discomfort.

Distance learning instruction in exercise or assessment may—or may not—be allowed depending on the location of the school or program and accrediting agencies. Schools and programs that wish to include online instruction should be up-to-date on regulatory requirements.

There is a possibility that tele-fitness and tele-rehabilitation will grow in popularity. If more clients opt for convenience of virtual instruction or want access to classes that are not offered locally, distance learning laboratory and practicum classes make sense. Teaching students how to navigate online instruction may provide them with useful skills for the workplace.

Managing the Virtual Classroom

A class is a temporary community that comes together for a defined period of time for the purposes of learning. Getting to know each other and staying on task helps students make connections and grow. Managing a virtual classroom is a bit different than a face-to-face course. This can be especially challenging when a student is enrolled in several different distance learning classes at the same time. When all of the classrooms look alike in the LMS it can be challenging to differentiate one classroom from another.

The combination of interactive and self-directed learning can create fuzzy boundaries for instructional time. Clear expectations and consistency throughout course activities are important to provide structure. The lack of opportunity for casual interaction leaves little opportunity for students to obtain answers to simple questions that could be asked while walking down a hallway after a face-to-face class. Frequent reminders about deadlines including posted announcements and review during live classes may seem excessive, but might be necessary to get students' attention.

Students who are new to distance learning may have difficulty understanding expectations regarding participation. Reaching out to students and reminding them what to do might be needed until they are able to navigate the course on their own. Instructors that balance communication by using a combination of leading strategies and active listening can serve as a model for what is expected of students. Building assessments into every activity requires students to participate. It provides opportunities to get feedback from students, give feedback to them, and get to know them.

Student Readiness

When students are new to a distance learning environment, assessing student readiness is important to set them up for success. The first step is providing general information so students can decide whether they are ready and able to enroll in a course or program. For students who opt to enroll, part of readiness includes providing information ahead of the course opening so they can plan, make purchases, and make adjustments if needed. Details should include information about the place, space, and time for course activities as well as any factors that are relevant to academic readiness.

Technology

Prior to enrolling in a distance learning course, students should be informed of the minimum technology requirements needed to engage with the course. This refers to the equipment needed and the student's ability to effectively use the equipment to participate in the class. Information about technology requirements should be provided on the institution or program website. This is likely applicable to all courses whether they are distance learning or not. Students who are considering enrolling have the opportunity to self-assess their technology and its capabilities.

A **computer** that is compatible with the LMS and any apps or programs required to read or produce course files. The computer should have an updated operating system and antivirus software. Many videoconferencing platforms and LMSs are compatible with smartphones. But students should not attempt to undertake a distance learning course using only a smartphone. This is especially important when students will be required to submit assignments that would be challenging to complete on a small screen. Tablets may be handy to view videos and access some areas of the LMS. But they may not be adequately equipped to store files or assignments.

A **webcam, headset, and microphone**. To minimize audio feedback, all participants in live sessions should use a headset instead of built in microphone and speakers. If courses will require students to be visible on camera when the course is in progress, students must be informed ahead of time so they can arrange space to be mindful of privacy (for family members and roommates) and background noise.

Reliable high speed internet access at home. Internet speed should be adequate to allow video conferencing. This can be problematic if family members or roommates are online at the same time. Students should not attempt to rely on free internet in public places except in an emergency (e.g. local power outage.)

Adequate digital storage. Local storage on the computer should be backed up regularly to avoid losing assignments and saved course materials. Students may need to be reminded to use flash drives, an external hard drive, or cloud storage. If cloud storage is used it should be password protected and secure to maintain privacy.

Backup plan. Students should prepare ahead of time with a plan for what they can do if some of their technology fails.

Technical support. Ability to troubleshoot technical problems—or access to someone who can help them is important. Schools may offer phone consultations specific to the LMS or required apps. But that would not be adequate for a student who could not get a webcam to work, had a computer crash, or was unable to open a file. Students can be encouraged to identify a computer savvy friend or bookmark contact information for a nearby computer support professional.

Learning Space and Time

For seated class activities including synchronous class meetings, study time, and completing assignments, students should establish one or more dedicated spaces. The space should provide the opportunity to work without distractions. When students are setting up their space they should consider lighting, noise, and possibility of interruption. Remind them to also pay attention to ergonomics in spaces where they will be sitting for long periods of time.

For class activities that involve movement or demonstration—especially when students need to be visible on webcam—a dedicated space should be identified. Students should assess safety of the space so it is free of any objects that could topple over or interfere with movement. When students are performing movements or doing demonstrations at home, they may need to move the webcam around to provide the instructor and class with adequate views of their work.

If students will be expected to demonstrate practice teaching of exercises, that will factor into the considerations for learning space and time. In addition to fitness equipment, they will need to have agreement from a person to serve as a client for demonstration purposes.

Establishing alternate learning spaces or creating flexible seating gives students options. The kitchen or dining room table might provide the best ergonomic to work on a writing assignment, but might be noisy if others live at home. So it might not be a good option during a live course sessions or around mealtimes. The bedroom could be the quietest place for reading, but might be too far from the WiFi router to stream a synchronous session. For course activities that involve movement, the area with the most potential could be an outdoor patio or the living room, both of which have high potential for interruptions. If the student needs to commandeer a room in the basement or rig up a desk in the garage, planning ahead of time would be essential.

Often students opt for distance learning because they need flexibility, but that may not always be an option depending upon the course or program. Students in a distance learning course that requires any synchronous participation will need to know the schedule of activities so they can plan. Recording courses for later playback is an option to give students access to material. But that works for lectures, not courses that involve engagement and active learning. Informing students about required meeting times can help them decide if they are ready to fully participate in a course and able to meet attendance requirements

When courses are unexpectedly moved online due to inclement weather or other reasons students may have difficulty attending live course sessions. A spouse or roommate may also need to work from home on the family computer. Young children may require supervision in their own online learning. The internet speed may not be adequate for multiple individuals in the same household to simultaneously stream video. To plan for the unexpected, schools and programs should have written guidelines and policies regarding attendance and make up work.

Academic Preparedness

Entry level programs in post-secondary education generally do not require students to have specialized knowledge or experience. Students are expected to possess skills and abilities to learn along with basic knowledge from common core subjects (language arts, mathematics, science.) It is expected that students learned to read, write, solve problems, and developed study habits during their previous educational experiences. Students in U.S. programs who graduated from international schools may be required to submit Test of English as a Foreign Language (TOEFL) scores for English language proficiency.

The overall design of a learning arc for an educational program progresses from foundational courses to applied and integrated material. In exercise science, fitness, and kinesiology, foundational knowledge in anatomy & physiology is needed in order to apply information to advanced courses. When anatomy & physiology is a prerequisite for another course, the aim is to ensure that students possess a certain level of knowledge needed to succeed in the later course. Completion of a prerequisite is not a guarantee that a student can recall material so review may be needed. During course orientation instructors can summarize prerequisite course material that students are expected to know. To help students recall material from a prerequisite course, a list of supplemental resources can be provided to use as reference.

Use of co-requisite courses in curriculum design helps to coordinate learning. Requiring students to enroll in a pair of courses simultaneously can be used to create a learning community with students and instructors. The flow of content from one course to another can help students to synthesize material. In distance learning co-requisite requirements can be useful to encourage students to make connections with one another. When they see the same names and faces in multiple classes it can be easier to build relationships, seek help, and offer support.

Student Self-Management

Students in all settings (face-to-face, hybrid, or distance learning) need to be responsible to manage time, set priorities, and meet deadlines. They also need to know when and how to ask for help if needed. Providing adequate information and orientation to the course can help students know what will be expected of them and when.

Some institutions utilize **learning contracts** for distance learning. A learning contract outlines responsibilities and expected behaviors for students. A learning contract dovetails with institutional policies and the syllabus by detailing requirements for attendance, participation, and outlining the qualifications for a passing grade. A learning contract may be executed upon enrollment in a program or required for every course in which a student enrolls.

A learning contract administered at the program/institutional level will have general information about responsibilities and expected behaviors. When a learning contract is written for a course, it includes details about specific activities in the course and the expectations for students. The language used in a learning contract is written so that a student's signature is an acknowledgement that they have been informed of—and understand—actions they will need to take to be successful in the course. While a signature on a learning contract is not a guarantee that a student will succeed in distance learning, it reinforces the recognition of the student's responsibility in a program or course. If a course or program does not use a learning contract, students should still be provided a summary of expected behaviors and policies as part of course orientation.

It is a good idea to use an **instructional formula** throughout a course for materials and activities to help students stay oriented with consistent organization. For example, for every unit/module all students are expected to read one book chapter and take a quiz prior to the class meeting and contribute to a discussion forum after the class prior to the conclusion of the unit/module. This regular instructional formula provides a routine that can be balanced by other types of instructional activities and assignments such as small group work, independent assignments, and tests.

Requests for Accommodations

If a course activity is not fully accessible to a specific student, accommodations will be necessary to meet that student's individual needs. Students with a physical disability, vision or hearing impairment, or learning disability may need adaptations to presentation of material, alternatives for assignments or assessments, extended time, or changes to the instructional environment. The accommodations should not change what the student learns, only how they learn.

In order to receive accommodations, students must self-identify as a person with a disability and self-advocate. Students may not necessarily understand their rights to accommodation. They may also not be familiar with the process to make a request for accommodation. Prior to the start of class all students should be provided with information on how to self-identify with a disability or make a request for accommodations.

Medical documentation is not required to substantiate a student's self-report of a disability. The self-report of a limitation is adequate. It is helpful when a student can identify accommodations that have been effective (or ineffective) to overcome barriers to learning. Supplemental reports (e.g. a 504 Plan or Individualized Education Plan) or other documentation may contain useful information. It is important to note that planning for any student who seeks accommodations is done on an individual basis.

Some institutions have dedicated departments with staff who work with students with disabilities. Students with disabilities can request accommodations or instructional support through these departments. These departments may also provide instructional support services. Staff members in these departments may be able to serve as a resource for instructors regarding course accessibility and/or accommodations. For programs that are not located at an institution that has a department for students with disabilities, processes should be put in place to assist students in making requests for accommodations.

Worth noting, requirements and procedures for accommodation in education are handled differently than requests for accommodations on a board or licensing examination. For examinations, a documented prior history of accommodations may support the request for a board or licensing examination. But generally additional information is required. Students who need—and are entitled to—accommodations will need to serve as their own advocates for learning and testing.

Readiness Checklist

Providing a distance learning readiness checklist for students can be helpful. At minimum this should include technology requirements. A more robust version can include fundamental information from the course syllabus.

- Computer with keyboard that meets operating system requirements and has antivirus software

- Software and apps to complete assignments (video recording, preparing slides or documents, citation manager, etc.)

- Backup plan in case computer fails

- Headset with microphone

- Working webcam

- High-speed internet access

- Contact information for tech savvy friend or family member and agreement that they may be contacted if needed

- Contact information for computer support professional

- Digital storage for assignments

- Backup digital storage for assignments

- Quiet learning space for seated class activities

- Quiet learning space for live online activities that is near an outlet to charge electronic devices

- Learning space visible on camera for classes involving movement and demonstration

- Special supplies needed for the class

- Review the schedule of live course meetings

- Requirements for attendance during live classes (i.e. visible on webcam)

- List of prerequisite courses or material to review

- Instructions should also be included to direct students who may need accommodations to the right place to make the request.

Orientation

Learning to navigate a physical classroom begins when young children enter school. Students are advised on appropriate dress, instructed on necessary supplies, told what to bring to class, where to hang their coat, and where to sit. The classroom environment becomes more familiar over time and students know what is expected of them in subsequent courses. Students need to learn how to navigate the virtual classroom and may need guidance to get oriented.

Orientation specific for distance learning is important to help students become familiar with environment and set them up for success. A general orientation can be given to all students prior to the start of a term. For each class, a specific orientation should be provided. A combination of asynchronous and synchronous orientation activities can be used to help students feel connected.

The LMS landing page can include links to prerecorded presentations that use screen capture to show examples of general tasks and features of the LMS. An instructor can also post orientation videos within a course that demonstrate instructional strategies that students will use in that course. Saving short orientation videos in a repository in the LMS can be helpful for students to access later on if they need a refresher.

Email instructions can be sent about a week prior to the course start date with information on how to access the LMS. Invite students to test the technology and include information on who they can contact if they have problems. Students who are new to distance learning or are new to an LMS often want to know what a course looks like. Giving them access to a sample course can help them get oriented but access to course materials and instructional activities should be restricted until the actual start date for the course. If students are given early access to a course they may try to jump ahead. Most LMSs allow instructors to show or hide course materials from view. Some LMSs allow instructors to schedule release of materials. It is essential that instructional activities begin on the official course start date, not early. That will help instructors with time management and ensure that students stay on track.

Part of orientation can include a discussion forum for students to introduce themselves to the rest of the class. This is a good way to begin creating a community. A general introductory paragraph can be used, but a more creative approach can promote a higher level of student engagement. The discussion prompt could ask students to provide a structured response to a short list of questions. Students could make and share a slide presentation with three slides: where they are from, why they are in class now, and what they hope to get out of class. They could also be asked to record short video introductions. These types of activities can be helpful if they will be used in the course for assignments. The introductions discussion forum provides a good opportunity for instructors to model organization of topics and threads.

Orientation can include ungraded activities like games and quizzes. These can serve a dual purpose by helping students to get acclimated to the LMS and as informal assessments. For courses that involve prerequisites, students may need to be reminded that they will need to recall and retrieve information from a previous course. Giving them the option to take an ungraded quiz can help them learn how to take a quiz and also recall material from prerequisite courses

When a course will require active engagement for students the concept should be emphasized in orientation. Collaboration methods and instructional strategies can be introduced by using an icebreaker. Assign students to small groups. Examples of icebreaker activities that set the stage for involvement and collaboration include:

- Ask groups to select a mascot that includes each group member's favorite color.

- Draw a tree with a branch representing each group member placed in order of their height.

- Create a group motto that utilizes initials from each group member.

Icebreaker activities should be structured to eliminate the possibility that a single student will complete a task on behalf of a group without involvement from other group members. For live sessions these types of activities can be used to learn to navigate breakout rooms and effectively manage time. For asynchronous instruction this can introduce managing conversations that involve a time lag and collaborating within the group to meet a deadline.

When activities that will be used in instructional strategies are introduced informally it helps students begin to recognize the process. Students can be assigned roles, given time to work as a group, and then asked to report back to the class to deliver something. This follows a basic interactive format for small-group active learning. Asking students to produce something and share it with the class shows them how to use the small group time effectively and avoid getting sidetracked. An orientation that introduces methods required for engagement to students also provides the opportunity for the instructor to practice facilitation.

Conversations between students, instructors, and administrators in distance learning need to take place at the right time and in the right place. Making a distinction between instructional conversations and administrative conversations helps everyone use time more effectively. Directing students to the appropriate communication pathway can help avoid frustration when they need help or an answer to a question.

Administrative conversations do not belong in course sessions. These can take place via phone call or via email. This applies to registration questions, requests for a registration over-ride or waiver of a prerequisite, and resolution of an incomplete grade or other grade dispute. Discussions about accommodations for students with disabilities should take place in a way that allows the conversations to be documented while maintaining confidentiality for the student.

Any questions or conversations about course material should take place in that course's area in the LMS. It is not uncommon for students to email instructors with questions. If not managed, this can turn into private tutoring via email. This places demands on the instructor's time and is not fair to other students who may need help with the same question. When students email with questions, redirecting students to post the question in the appropriate area on the course page allows other students to hear the question and review the answer. Instructors may need to repeatedly redirect students who reach out for instructional help via email.

Communication Pathways

Including general Q&A forums can provide a place for students to ask general questions. Creating a **help forum** that is positioned at the top of the course page near the syllabus and announcements provides a place for students to ask questions outside of the current course unit or module. This can be interactive allowing other students to answer or contribute to a discussion thread.

A **general questions forum** can be included in each module to provide a space to promote informal conversations about that module. If it is designed as an open forum students can start a discussion thread in addition to responding to other questions or comments. This can encourage students to synthesize material as the course progresses by providing space for students to share thoughts separately from instructional material.

Incorporating non-instructional forums for help or general questions can encourage students to interact with each other which promotes a sense of community. Training students to use the right pathway for communication takes patience. This is especially important when students are used to private communication with instructors or carry on tangential conversations in an instructional forum.

Virtual Student Lounge

Part of the experience of being a student is gathering informally with other students. For face-to-face courses this happens organically before and after class when students are in the same space. The physical space of a campus generally has lounges or gathering places for students, staff, and instructors to have casual conversations. It creates a sense of belonging and provides opportunities to learn about—and from—each other.

In distance learning **a virtual student lounge** can be created to provide similar opportunities for connections. Ideally the virtual student lounge can be housed in the LMS so that it can be accessed from within the virtual instructional environment. This maintains a connection with the school and allows a level of monitoring.

A virtual student lounge hosted on the LMS is an equivalent of being on school grounds. This creates a connection with the school. It provides the potential for oversight by the school or program that does not exist in an unmonitored social media group. That would be important if conflict between students arose or if material was perceived as inappropriate. Providing a format that fosters a sense of belonging can help promote student engagement.

In some cases creation of a virtual student lounge may be beyond technological capabilities of a school or program. If that is the case a social media group can be set up that is hosted by the school or program. This provides an online gathering space that is connected to the school.

A virtual student lounge can provide an informal place for instructors, administrators, and students to communicate and share information. Discussion forums can be used for introductions, special interest groups, and exchange of resources. With permission, results of student projects can be shared—much in the same way a binder of a thesis might be placed in administrative offices for casual perusal.

Encouraging Collaboration

Collaboration is essential for group project-based learning. It is not uncommon for students to attempt to circumvent collaboration by taking a divide-and-conquer approach to the project. The result is often a product that resembles Frankenstein's monster (multiple disconnected parts) rather than something coherent and cohesive. Students may need to be encouraged and guided to effectively collaborate with each other.

Collaborative activities and assignments can be structured to require students to take on different roles—each of which requires a different type of participation. This can foster a sense of belonging to the group. It also helps students take collective ownership of a project. For team-based learning or just in time instruction, students can be assigned roles as facilitator, recorder, timekeeper, or researcher. This provides structure to the group and allows students to select a role that seems natural to them.

Using the same types of small group activities on a regular basis can be helpful. Students become familiar with the process so they know what to expect. When they understand the format it can help them find ways to navigate within their group. If the same type of activity is used multiple times with the membership of the small groups reconfigured each time, it helps students develop communication and collaboration skills.

Creating a Civil Environment

Guidelines for distance learning should include ground rules about etiquette for both synchronous and asynchronous communication. This can be as general as reminding everyone to take turns speaking and listening respectfully. If students are required to be visible on camera, they may need to be reminded to be properly clothed. Everyone likely will need to be reminded to mute microphones when not presenting or speaking.

Students may log into synchronous class sessions from unusual places or noisy environments. This is not necessarily disrespectful. Nor is it always an indication that the student is disinterested or not paying attention. Rather it can be mean that the student is unable to find a quiet place or is managing competing priorities. A student attending class from bed wearing pajamas might be in the quietest place in their home. If the student's background environment is consistently disruptive or interferes with participation in synchronous sessions, the instructor may need to schedule an advisement session to inform the student and strategize alternatives.

Allowing time for general Q&A at designated times in live classes maximizes instructional time. Following a process to field live questions can help students know when it they can have a turn speaking. Some platforms have a feature allowing a student to raise a virtual hand. If that is not the case, students could raise their hand on webcam and be called on by the instructor to unmute their microphone to ask a question. In large classes students can be asked to type questions into the course chat or directed to a question forum in the LMS. The latter may be an easier option for instructors to manage and students to track.

Discussion forums and course chat can be tricky to moderate. The modern era of text message and social media has made short comments, sentence fragments, and use of emojis socially acceptable. To a degree, that has shaped perceptions for what is appropriate for conversations in a virtual environment. Abrupt comments, flippant responses, or derogatory remarks are poorly received in a written setting when there is no opportunity to deflect, clarify, or smooth things over. This can spark arguments and escalate into unfortunate interactions.

To encourage students to be polite, respectful, and thorough, they can be asked to write in paragraphs when they contribute to a discussion forum. Students should be informed—and reminded—that anything they say in the classroom should be thoughtfully and professionally put forth. Encourage them to defend their position rather than simply state an opinion. Students may also need to be reminded to "listen" to others in the class by making sure they review responses in a discussion forum before making a contribution. Instructors should constantly monitor discussion forums and have a system to intervene if necessary.

Privacy and Confidentiality

Privacy is freedom from unwanted attention or scrutiny. Confidentiality is a way to maintain privacy by preventing unwanted or unauthorized disclosure. Selection of instructional tools and methods of instruction must take privacy and confidentiality into account. This permits academic freedom. Instructors can introduce challenging topics. Students can ask silly questions. A class can engage in debate on difficult topics without fear of retaliation or misinterpretation. While students are learning and exploring they have a right to privacy in the classroom. It is important that instructors and students must honor privacy and confidentiality for course participants.

Students and instructors must know who has **access to their course** at any given time. For a face-to-face class it is easy to see when a visitor is in the classroom. Virtual classrooms are different. Access to the LMS or videoconference sessions should be restricted to instructors and students. When others are given access to a course, students should be informed. If guests are involved in distance learning classes they should be allowed in to the learning space for a defined period of time and then excused once the participation has ended. The same is true for administrators or colleagues who may be charged with observation of instructors.

Tech support staff often have access to courses for the purposes of providing help if needed. Depending upon how the LMS is configured, these individuals may be visible to students—or not. Tech support staff may never need to enter a course. If they do, students should be informed of their presence and their role in supporting the course.

In a face-to-face class, anything said in the classroom remains in the classroom. Once the class is over the instructor and student walk out the door and there is no permanent record of any of the discussion. Distance learning is different because digital records are created as part of course discussion forums, materials submitted for assignments, and recorded sessions. All of these materials should stay within the course, just like material for a physical classroom. When class sessions are recorded, access to the recording should be restricted to the class. Students may benefit from reviewing sessions. A student who missed a session can "attend" at a later time. To ensure privacy of all participants, contributions to discussion forums, materials submitted for assignments, and any recordings of class sessions should not be shared or distributed to anyone outside of the course without permission.

Academic Integrity

Questions about academic integrity often surface during discussions about distance learning. Specifically in regard to how an instructor can ensure that the student is doing his or her own work. Two ways to address academic integrity are policies and getting to know the students.

Policies regarding academic integrity should be part of the distance-learning experience. These should clearly indicate what is expected of students in terms of respect, honesty, and responsibility. The process for investigating possible violations of academic integrity should be outlined as well as the penalties for violation.

For tests and quizzes, if proctoring is to be used students should be informed at the beginning of the course. If proctoring involves video recordings of students taking an assessment, the recordings should be preserved for the duration of time that any student can appeal that assessment or the grade for the course. If resource materials are permitted during a test or quiz, adequate care should be taken in the delivery to create the test environment to enable students to use the permitted materials efficiently and effectively.

Plagiarism is a problem throughout education. Students can knowingly—or unknowingly—use another author's work without proper acknowledgement or citation. Most academic institutions impose serious penalties for cheating—including plagiarism. Teaching students about plagiarism, how to cite material that is sourced from someplace else, and how to utilize resources in order to put forth their own original thoughts can all help to combat plagiarism. Originality software programs (Turn

It In) and general internet searches can identify material that is not original to the student.

Instructors can get to know the students in distance learning when they engage with them. For synchronous distance learning, instructors and students can see and hear each other using videoconferencing technology. Through the visual connection it is accepted that the person attending the class is the student who is involved in course activities and interactions (e.g. presentations, videos, discussions.)

Incorporating low stakes writing activities during the course (e.g. discussion forums, short papers) can help instructors learn each student's written voice and writing style. When low stakes writing is used to scaffold a larger assignment (e.g. case study, research paper) it can provide ongoing instructional activity. Students can learn how to leverage reference material, cite properly, and organize their ideas into a manuscript while minimizing the chance that a student would use someone else's work for a single high stakes writing assignment.

A number of websites allow anyone to hire a writer for a nominal fee for a writing a paper or creating a project. If material is submitted for an assigned activity in a voice that significantly differs from the student's voice or clearly sourced from somewhere else the instructor can address that with the student.

Time Management

There is a perception that distance learning requires more time for instructors than teaching face-to-face classes. All types of teaching involve preparation, instructional time, and grading. But online teaching also requires troubleshooting technology problems when they arise. If instructors do not make an effort to organize course activities, extra time may be needed to provide feedback to—or meet with—individual students. This can place excessive demands on the instructor's time.

Stage Interactions

Using staged interactions can save time and promote student engagement by providing facilitated opportunities for communication and informal assessments. Mini presentations by individual students or small groups can infuse instruction with fresh energy and provide opportunities for students to apply course concepts. Collaborative assignments that use a report back from groups to the whole class provide the opportunity for students to learn from each other. After staged interactions, when the instructor takes time to refine information or clarify concepts it gives students feedback and can help to create a learning arc.

Minimize Volume

Worksheets, short answer essays, and other types of recall assignments require individual attention to each student when instructors grade and give feedback. The purpose of these assignments is often to demonstrate that students comprehend information. But the time demands for manually grading a large volume of these types of assignments can be overwhelming. Substituting online quizzes for these types of assignments provides a similar type of assessment. When **automatic grading** is used for quizzes or tests, students get instant feedback and it saves time. Once all students have taken the quiz or test the instructor can review the grades and identify content areas for which the class could benefit from additional review. This information can be used like the Just in Time instructional strategy to focus the instruction in the class following completion of the quiz or test.

Another option to minimize volume is to incorporate worksheets, essays, or other assignments into instructional activities in a flipped classroom. Students have a learning experience when they complete an activity prior to class. Repurposing the material to use during a live class session provides the student with feedback during the activity and eliminate the need for the instructor to grade individual assignments.

Scaffold Large Projects

Scaffolding or using a tiered approach to larger assignments by breaking them into smaller parts can be an effective way to maximize time and feedback. The smaller activities can be assessed as the larger project is constructed. For example, require students to submit different parts of a research paper (e.g. selection of topic, resource list, methods) as they work. This creates a flow of formative feedback and helps students stay on track. It also enables instructors to become familiar with each student's work. That familiarity can make final grading of large assignments less onerous because the instructor will know what to expect.

Set Boundaries

It is not unusual for instructors who are new to distance learning to feel overwhelmed with different types of activities and multiple communication pathways. Depending upon how synchronous class time is structured it may not provide adequate opportunities to answer all questions or provide advisement to students.

BEYOND LECTURES

When assignments and asynchronous activities are incorporated into a class, the students may be engaged with a course in evenings or on weekends. If that is when instructors schedule "time off" there can be a lag in communication. Reconfiguring the online work environment by setting boundaries for questions and consultations helps to keep work and communication organized.

Instructors can easily feel that they are on duty 24 hours a day, 7 days per week if they are preparing instructional activities, grading assessments, checking emails, and reviewing/monitoring asynchronous course activities. It can be helpful to establish a timeline for grading assignments and giving feedback to students so the students know what to expect. Reviewing and responding to discussion forums at regularly scheduled time can be useful for instructors to manage time and to give students an idea of when they will hear from the instructor.

Manage Communication

In face-to-face classes, sometimes students will approach the instructor after class to ask a question. They may be seeking a connection, afraid to speak up in class, or expect individualized attention. Distance learning is not all that different. When an instructor immediately responds to email, students may view that communication pathway as a faster way to get an answer. Training students at the beginning of class can be a good start. If email questions persist, gentle reminders with directions may be needed:

> "That is a very good question. No doubt other students have the same question. Would you please post this to the current discussion forum

[or the help forum] in the course? I can answer it there. It will help everyone—especially other students who might be afraid to ask."

Orient students—and remind them—where to initiate questions about the course or course material. Schedule a dedicated time each day to read and respond to questions. Let students know the schedule to give them an idea when they can expect an answer. This will help them feel heard and not abandoned if an answer is not provided immediately.

Office Hours and Appointments

In higher education, office hours are a dedicated time that faculty members are scheduled to be in their offices and available to students for help or advisement. For instructors in distance learning, scheduling online office hours can help time management and facilitate communication with students. The instructor can log into videoconferencing at a regular time every week and invite students to drop in for a synchronous meeting. Office hours are appropriate for general discussions and group help because anyone can drop in. Therefore multiple students may be present in the conference at the same time. When a private conversation with a student is needed it should not take place during office hours if others can drop in. An appointment for a conference should be scheduled on a separate line (e.g. Skype, Google Hangouts, etc.) that limits access to the instructor and student to ensure confidentiality.

Assessment and Feedback

In some educational settings, assessments are designed to be punitive. High stakes tests, harsh grading, and criticism can be disheartening for students. Penalties for missed classes, late assignments, or poor grades can cause struggling students to fall behind. Rather than serving as an incentive for students to try harder, assessments can be a disincentive. In exercise and fitness education, anatomy & physiology provides a good example. Students may try to rely on memorization (for the purposes of passing multiple choice examinations) rather than learning the material (to apply it later.) Short term memorization techniques can make it difficult to retain information and apply concepts. This approach may not provide the student with a foundation that will be needed for hands-on courses and clinical reasoning.

When assessments can be designed to get and give feedback about learning, a course can feel more collaborative. Ongoing assessment can help instructors find out if the class is struggling with specific content areas, tasks, or skills. This can identify need for review of material or further exploration of a topic. Incorporating a variety of different types of assessments can provide a more holistic picture of student engagement and progress. Students are likely to be more motivated when they have ongoing feedback on their progress. After all, their job as students is to learn.

Assessment in any course should take place on an ongoing basis throughout the course. Frequent assessments help instructors identify when content or concepts need to be reviewed or revised. Students in distance learning can have difficulty feeling connected and motivated. Because assessments require students to contribute and includes feedback from instructors, any assessment gives them a chance for connection. Students can self-monitor their progress and recognize when/if to seek instructional support.

Types of Assessments

Because licensing and certification requirements rely on minimum contact hours and multiple choice examinations, it is all too easy for courses to follow the same (un-engaging) format of lectures and tests. Visibility on webcam during a live course meeting is an easy way to track attendance to meet contact hour requirements. But it is not a measure of engagement. Frequent use of multiple choice tests can familiarize students with the format of a licensing or certification examination. But it does not adequately capture learning. Assessments of student learning during a course is different than program evaluation. Instructors should identify opportunities for assessments that encourage student learning and monitor student progress in ways that align with course objectives.

Attendance and Participation

Attendance in class is showing up. Participation is engagement. Attendance is not the same as participation. This is especially relevant in distance learning—and for programs that require a minimum number of contact hours. Students should be informed of requirements for attendance and participation in the syllabus and during orientation.

Attendance is measured by contact hours when a student is in the presence of an instructor during class time. This is part of the rationale to have live online lectures: students are present in the instructional environment and perhaps are visible on webcam. But because there are many other ways to actually engage students in distance learning, assessment of attendance needs to be configured to take student engagement with a course into account.

For courses that have attendance requirements, student engagement must be measured. Monitoring attendance can use a multifaceted approach when it is not based on live contact hours. Instructional design for distance learning can take into account how different interactions count as involvement in a course. Activities should be documented in some way so that the student workload can be assessed.

Depending upon the LMS or configuration, the instructor can see a student logged into the course, what areas of the course they visited, and for how long. If students are required to access learning materials, instructors can perform a quantitative assessment by auditing if and when students were in the appropriate area(s) of the LMS. For discussion forums, it is popular to require students to make a certain number of contributions. These contributions can also be counted.

Students who fall short of minimum attendance requirements generally are required to make up the time. For live course meetings, this often involves attending a different class for an equivalent amount of time. Other live class sessions must be available for the student to virtually attend, but they may not cover the same material. Another way to make up for missed attendance is requiring a student to submit an assignment that covers the missed material. This places an extra burden on instructors who must come up with a special assignment and review or grade it to assess whether the student met learning objectives for the missed session. It also can provide an incentive for students who do not wish to attend class but are happy to complete an assignment. For attendance that is measured by number of contributions to discussion forums, students who fall short may be asked to increase their level of participation in a subsequent unit or module.

It is fairly easy to see from these examples that monitoring attendance is not necessarily the most optimal way to assess a distance learning course. While monitoring attendance is important to ensure that students are showing up to class, assessments of participation and performance provide more insight into engagement, learning, and progress.

Participation in class can be measured several different ways. On a basic level it can be by counting the number of contributions a student makes in a class. Students can be required to fill out participation logs by recording when they participated in a discussion or learning activity and what they said or did. Instructors can review the logs on a regular basis. Ongoing self-evaluation can help students reflect on how they are participating in the course and what they are accomplishing.

In terms of attendance and participation, face-to-face classes are different from distance learning. It is easier to measure attendance in a face-to-face class than participation. It is easier to measure participation in a distance learning class than attendance. The LMS maintains records on when students access the course and complete course activities. So when attendance and participation are part of a course grade methods should be established for assessment.

Academic Performance

Assessments of academic performance are measurements of student knowledge, skills, or abilities relevant to course goals and material. A range of different tools can be used for assessment. Quizzes and examinations can be set up in the LMS for students to take online. These generally can accommodate different types of questions: multiple choice, matching, completion, true/false, short answer, and essay. Depending upon the design, they can be automatically graded to provide students with immediate feedback and save time for instructors. Worksheets, games, collaborative assignments, projects, and other activities can be structured to assess academic performance and offer more flexibility to be used for targeted feedback to students. Overall, assessment can be separated into three basic categories: informal, formative, and summative.

An **informal assessment** is an activity where the instructor provides an evaluation of student work without assigning a grade. Informal assessments can be planned or spontaneous and interspersed in teaching activities. They can include polls, reflections, or evaluations of active learning sessions or feedback from students. The rather ubiquitous "are there any questions?" is an informal assessment because it offers students the opportunity volunteer course content or instructional procedures that require clarification. In distance learning, feedback sought during live sessions, in online discussions, or through course chat serves as informal assessment. Instructors can use informal assessments to change instructional strategies or update course content if needed.

Formative assessments are graded quizzes, tests, or assignments that take place at intervals throughout a course. Typically many smaller formative assessments are used as lower-stakes assessments so that they provide an evaluation but do not substantially influence the student's grade in a course. Formative assessments can be used to chart student progress. Requiring students to include an explanation of their thought process to arrive at an answer provides an opportunity for metacognition. When they reflect on what they learn and how they learn that can help them revise study strategies (if needed.) Strategically timed formative assessments help students recognize that learning can improve over time. When different types of formative assessments are used in a course it can provide a more conducive learning environment for students with different learning preferences.

Summative assessments are measurements of knowledge, skills, or abilities at the end of a unit, course, or program. These are cumulative assessments that measure overall understanding. Summative assessment are often high stakes meaning they can have a large impact on a student's grade in a course. Midterm and final exams are summative assessments. Project-based learning (e.g. research paper) can also be used for summative assessments when the final product is evaluated as a major component of the course grade. When courses rely solely on summative assessments students do not receive feedback on their progress in time to remediate (if necessary.) This is an important consideration in distance learning if students feel lost without direct contact and support from other students.

Ideally a combination of formative and summative assessments can be used in a course to provide information on progress and demonstrate mastery of material. Charting out the formative and summative assessments can help instructors and students recognize and appreciate the learning arc for a course.

Competency

In **competency-based education**, students are assessed on knowledge, skills, and abilities, not only the amount of time spent in class. Attendance and contact hours are not entirely relevant because students can spend more or less time working to achieve learning outcomes. However, competency-based education is not simply self-study to pass a challenge exam. Rather it is a framework that identifies specific tasks or benchmarks that allow the student to demonstrate achievement or proficiency in knowledge, skill or ability.

When a student is able demonstrate competency early in the course, (s)he does not simply pass the course. Rather, participation in the course continues providing the student with the opportunity to demonstrate consistent demonstration of a skill/ability, further improvement of the skill/ability, and even application of advanced concepts. If a student takes longer to achieve proficiency than others in the class, all students are still learning and participating—just at different levels. Competency-based assessment allows for the possibility of remediation for a student who meets contact hour requirements, but does not meet benchmarks or is unable to demonstrate proficiency.

In exercise science and personal training education, practicum or internship provide good examples. Students would be required to attend a minimum number of hours, lead a certain number of sessions, and maybe write a paper or pass a test on relevant content. A basic assessment in this scenario would include attendance, observation by the preceptor, and grades on activities and/or projects.

Competency based assessment would look a little bit different. All of the same activities would be used, but students could be assessed for achievement of benchmarks and consistency in meeting those benchmarks. They could be assessed on their ability to efficiently conduct a client interview, confidently conduct assessments, and creatively design sessions to meet client needs. Assessment on an ongoing basis would help identify areas of achievement as well as opportunities for improvement.

In some ways competency based assessment provides a clearer picture of a learning arc than assessments based on academic achievement. For programs and instructors, the subjective and qualitative aspects of competency-based assessment may actually be uncomfortable, especially with a student population that is achievement-oriented and working towards a grade. It can be helpful to create detailed rubrics that clearly outline expectations, domains of assessment, and different levels of proficiency/achievement.

Peer Grading

Peer grading is used in different contexts for students to assess each other's work. A common way peer grading is used is to require students to exchange papers, tests, or assignments to review and grade. Instructors often do this to promote honesty—so students do not change answers when the class grades an assessment. It can also be a learning activity when the assessment is reviewed with the entire class.

Another way peer grading is used is by asking students in group or collaborative activities to evaluate each other. Asking students to grade each other's work or performance in a learning activity can be perilous. Personalities, friendships, and/or disagreements can factor into peer grading in this context. This can unfairly penalize or reward students when the grade based on something other than performance.

The ability to rate another student's comment or contribution to a discussion forum can help students connect online. A "like" or a "star" can be a simple indication that they are listening to each other. But it may also be considered a form of peer grading depending on how the instructor uses the ratings. Instructors should be transparent with students about how ratings (if applicable) factor into grading of student work.

Self-Assessment

Self-assessment is considered an important aspect of adult learning. Students can recognize their achievements and identify areas/strategies for improvement. Self-assessment promotes reflection and can help with motivation. Participation, engagement, and self-management provide good opportunities for self-assessment in distance learning. Examples of questions that could be used for self-assessment include:

- My contributions to discussions showed that I was prepared.

- I referenced course materials in my answers or comments.

- I was able to find and utilize supplemental resource material to support my contributions.

- My responses indicated that I listened to others in the class and acknowledged their feedback.

Students could be asked to rate responses to these types of questions using a Likert scale (never, rarely, sometimes, usually, always.) If the same self-assessment is completed again at different times during a course it can be used to help the students recognize improvement.

Self-assessments can also be used for collaborative or group activities. Students can be asked to describe their major contribution(s) to a group assignment and state the percent that their effort contributed to the overall activity. This can be a more constructive approach than having students assign grades to each other. The results of this type of assessment can be insightful for instructors—especially if the burden of a group assignment is not equally shared by all group members.

Multiple assessments of different values that are spaced throughout a course provide a broader picture of student progress than a single summative assessment. Different methods of assessments and timing can identify targeted areas for individual students that require improvement.

Selection of assessments should take desired learning outcomes and objectives in mind.

Creating and Using Rubrics

A rubric is a scoring guide that can be used to evaluate and score student work or progress. Categories that outline expectations for the assignment or learning activity are cross referenced with a score or evaluation of the student's performance. Rubrics can be designed to include space for individualized feedback to students to identify what they did well and areas that need improvement.

Different types of rubrics include: holistic, analytic, single point. These can be used as general or assignment specific assessments. General rubrics that include a combination of qualitative and quantitative assessments can be designed to measure things like participation or professionalism. Assignment specific rubrics can be developed for various class activities.

Instructors can evaluate students using a rubric, or students can be asked to complete their own rubric for self-reflection. Providing the grading rubric to students prior to the activity can be helpful for them to see how their work will be evaluated. When rubrics are used for graded activities, numerical ratings are assigned to include an overall score in addition to qualitative feedback.

Holistic Rubrics

Holistic rubrics provide an overall assessment on a single scale. These typically contain 3 to 5 different levels of performance or proficiency with a score attached to each level. The description of the criteria for each level generally includes several characteristics. Students need to meet all aspects of that level in order to receive the grade.

Holistic rubrics can be completed quickly by instructors and can be used to provide general insights. However, they do not provide targeted feedback to each student. Students may need additional feedback from the instructor that identifies ways they can improve their performance or work towards proficiency.

The following example of a holistic rubric for course participation has four levels; description for each scoring level includes three different criteria: visibility, relevance of questions or comments, and engagement. In this example, scoring for a student who was visibly present, highly engaged, but consistently off topic would fall into different categories. In order to provide higher quality information for the student to improve performance, the instructor would need to provide feedback in addition to a rating.

Table 1: Example of a Holistic Rubric

Score	Criteria
4	Visibly present in class. Consistently offered insights or asked astute questions appropriate to learning activity and content. Highly engaged with instructor and others in class.
3	Generally present in class. Most questions or comments were appropriate to learning activity and content. Moderate level of engagement with instructor and others.
2	Visible in class enough to meet minimum attendance requirement. Asked questions that were off topic or not relevant to current learning activity. Responsive to instructor but not to other students.
1	Limited visibility in class. Rarely answered or asked questions. Little engagement with instructor or others.

Single Point Rubrics

When the aim of an assessment is to give balanced, qualitative feedback to students a single point rubric can be used. This type has 3 to 5 different categories or domains as criteria for assessment. For each there is space to provide a targeted assessment of student performance on each criteria. The specific expectations for performance are not provided making this an individualized assessment.

The name "single point" can be misleading. The "point" refers to each specific criteria rather than a numerical point. If a single point rubric is used only for qualitative feedback and does not have a numerical scale attached it can be difficult to include as part of the course grade. Single point rubrics work very well as self-assessments by students. When included as part of the course grade, it can simply be marked as a complete assignment.

The following example of a single point rubric identifies different criteria for participation. It does not specify an expected level of performance. This is expanded from the holistic rubric to show how additional criteria can be included for evaluation and feedback.

Single point rubrics can be time consuming because instructors need to write targeted feedback for each student. Depending upon how the rubric is designed, this can feel monotonous. A benefit of using single point rubrics is that each student can get insight into what they can improve. This can be useful for competency based assessments. It can be helpful for instructors when a course has students with different levels of experience or academic preparedness.

Table 2: Example of a Single Point Rubric

Criteria	Assessment
Presence and visibility in class	*Strengths* *Areas for Improvement*
Engagement with instructor and classmates	*Strengths* *Areas for Improvement*
Preparation for course meetings and discussions	*Strengths* *Areas for Improvement*
Inclusiveness and respect	*Strengths* *Areas for Improvement*

Analytic Rubrics

Analytic rubrics can be used to provide a combination of an overall and targeted assessment. This type of rubric includes different criteria for assessment that are cross referenced with performance ratings or grade categories. The level of detail provided gives students the opportunity to recognize what is expected to achieve different levels of performance. This can be helpful for students who need to improve on certain criteria but not others.

When numerical scores are assigned to each criteria and performance level, an overall score can be calculated. This can be used in the same way as a holistic rubric to give each student an overall picture. If a numerical score is not used, the instructor can check or circle an assessment for the student in each category. Additional qualitative feedback can also be provided. Analytic rubrics can be time consuming to create, but can be completed relatively quickly.

The following example of an analytic rubric for participation uses four criteria and three different performance ratings. For each criterion specific information is included regarding expectations for different levels of performance. A basic grading scale is included to show how a distribution of grades for the class could be calculated. Since each performance level includes a range, it is be helpful for instructors to provide some rationale for assignment of points to identify areas for improvement.

Table 3: Example of an Analytic Rubric

Criteria	Assessment
Presence in class ___pts.	Visibly present in class and attentive to the discussions. (20-25 pts.)
	Meet minimum attendance requirements. (15-19 pts.)
	Limited visibility in class. (0-14 pts.)
Engagement ___pts.	Consistently offer insights or ask astute questions appropriate to learning activity and content. (20-25 pts.)
	Ask questions that are off topic or not relevant to current learning activity. (15-19 pts.)
	Little interaction with instructor or others. (0-14 pts.)
Preparation ___pts.	Use materials to effectively prepare for participation in class meetings or discussions. (20-25 pts.)
	Generally complete pre-work. Occasionally lack adequate preparation for participation. (15-19 pts.)
	Incomplete work or late assignments interfere with ability to participate in class. (0-14 pts.)
Respect ___pts.	Demonstrate willingness to listen to different opinions and ideas. (20-25 pts.)
	Some difficulty accepting opinions or ideas. (15-19 pts.)
	Resistant to information or opinions of others. (0-14 pts.)

Total points: _____

Giving Feedback

On a fundamental level, feedback is information provided to someone to let them know how they are doing. Feedback may include praise, criticism, evaluation, or assessment that helps the recipient of the feedback recognize areas for improvement. As students are developing and honing skills and abilities, feedback helps them know when they are on the right track. In order to be effective, feedback should be timely, instructional, specific, and sensitive to the needs of each student.

The contents of feedback and the way in which it is given can affect how the student responds. Feedback should be linked to learning objectives for the overall course or to a specific instructional activity. Feedback and a critique are not the same thing. A critique focuses on negative aspects of performance or behavior. Feedback can help the student identify what they are doing well and what they can improve. Depending upon the process to give feedback to students it may also include a strategy for remediation or improvement.

Feedback can be given verbally or in writing. When feedback is verbal, students have the opportunity to ask questions or seek clarifications. A conversational approach can feel more personalized, but instructors should keep notes of what was said so the information can be used to track student progress later. Feedback can be provided in writing using a short summary or rubric. To foster a connection with students, they can be invited to write a brief response, acknowledgement, and/or an action plan to address needs for improvement. Using a framework to provide feedback can be helpful to ensure instructors are thorough and consistent in the information they provide to students. Different feedback models can be used to provide a framework.

Sandwich Feedback Model

For instructors who are uncomfortable giving feedback the sandwich feedback model is popular. This involves two positive comments that act like bookends around a critical evaluation or identification of a need for improvement. A goal of the sandwich model is to provide ample opportunity to give praise or positive assessments. An example of this model to give a student feedback on participation in a role play that was used for an observational learning activity:

- I know you were reluctant to be the first student to participate in the clinic role-play activity. But you did a good job trying to come up with interview questions. (Praise)

- The case scenario upon which the role play was based contained details on risk factors and symptoms. Some of this essential information was missing from your questions. It would have helped you conduct a more robust interview. Make sure underline or highlight information in the case scenarios as you study. That will help you learn to ask more thorough questions. (Critical Evaluation)

- Thank you for demonstrating active listening skills. It shows evidence that you watched the videos on communication skills. (Praise)

There are plusses and minuses to the sandwich approach. It is best suited to identify a single area for improvement, not a strategy for remediation. If a student is struggling to meet performance goals, it may be difficult to find areas to praise. Inclusion of positive information can help soften criticism.

Wrap Feedback Model

A wrap feedback model can be used to obtain or give feedback. When it is used in education it actively engages the student by emphasizing action-oriented feedback and encouraging them to take ownership of their learning. The wrap model has five parts: context, observations, feelings, value, and suggestions for improvement.

Context can be used to link the feedback to the learning objectives for the activity. Observation is a summary of the student's performance. Feelings are a qualitative assessment of student engagement. Value is how the student applies what they have learned. Suggestions for improvement are next steps the student can take to improve their performance. Feedback on a role play activity using a wrap model might look something like the following example.

- This was our third role play demonstration in class. It required you and your partner to model an interview on a more complicated topic than the previous demonstrations. (Context)

- You clearly focused the conversation around back pain. That was the client's primary problem. Narrowing the discussion to musculoskeletal overlooked the potential for other risk factors associated with acute or chronic back pain. (Observations)

- I feel you did a good job thinking on your feet and modeling a professional conversation. (Feelings)

- Back pain is a common problem. Learning how to ask questions in an interview with a client will be very useful in your future practice. (Value)

- It would be a good idea to review the material on back pain to identify questions or assessments that would be good additions to an interview with a client. (Suggestions)

A wrap feedback model makes for a longer conversation with students. But it can be a framework for a more thoughtful discussion that taps into actions the student can take to work towards improvements. A benefit of this model is the inclusion of context. This can remind students of learning objectives and expected performance outcomes associated with the course.

Chronological Model

The chronological model of giving feedback reviews the learning activity in sequence from beginning to end. The instructor provides a commentary on what went well and what could have been better. Key benchmarks in the activity are used as focal points in the summary to follow the arc of the activity from beginning, to middle, and end. This approach can be made more student-centered by inviting them to review and reflect by asking them to explain what they were thinking or feeling at key points in the activity. Chronological feedback given for a practice client interview could look like the following example.

- The role play started out smoothly. You started with a professional greeting and asked some good questions. The client had some difficulty answering these initial questions. What other questions might you have asked? (Beginning)

- In the middle of the role play you asked some good questions about daily activities that caused discomfort for the client. How could you have been more specific? Could you have incorporated some functional movement assessments?

- At the end of the role play you struggled with summarizing what you learned and outlining a plan. Can you describe what barriers you felt?

The chronological approach works well when a learning activity is recorded. The instructor and student(s) can review the recording together. The recording can be paused at critical points to provide opportunity for discussion.

A benefit of the chronological model is that it provides students with the opportunity to replay the activity. This can be useful to review decisions and consider alternate approaches to the activity. A difficulty with the chronological model is that it is time consuming to execute. If the activity is not graded, the feedback may be useful but the students may be unsure how to use the feedback in relation to other assessments that are part of the course grade.

Pendleton's Approach to Feedback

The Pendleton approach to feedback uses open ended questions and observations to guide the student to an action plan. This approach, sometimes called

Pendleton's rules, includes a combination of positive information and critical evaluation of what went well and what needs improvement. A benefit of this model is that it includes opportunities for the student to self-reflect. This can serve to help students become more engaged in the feedback conversation. It can also encourage them to reflect on how they approach learning (metacognition.) The following example follows Pendleton's approach for feedback on a practice client interview.

- What do you think went well for you in this role play? (Question to prompt reflection)

- Your confidence has improved since the last role play session. This time you were able to think on your feet and ask follow up questions to elicit information from your partner. (Observation of what went well.)

- What would you do differently next time? (Ideas for an action plan)

- To help organize your thoughts, try taking a few moments to review the client's file before starting the interview. That can help you streamline your questions to focus on important information that requires clarification. (Suggestion for what to do differently next time.)

The questions in this model can be general (e.g. "What went well?") or structured with specific prompts (e.g. "How did you structure the interview to obtain important information from your partner in the practice role play?") Instructors should plan to use questions that are aligned with the learning objectives for the activity.

Students can be encouraged to take notes immediately after they receive feedback. This can promote self-reflection and help to solidify the action plan.

STAR Feedback Model

The STAR model acronym makes it easy to remember. This model is an outline to provide structured feedback. Situation (S) and task (T) give instructors the opportunity to provide context for the feedback. Action (A) is a summary of what the student did—or said—in the activity. This can include positive or negative comments. Results (R) is what the student achieved in response to what they did during the activity. The following provides an example of the STAR model used to give feedback from a role play activity.

- You and your partner just conducted your first practice interview. (Situation)

- The objective of the activity was to ask follow up questions to clarify or expand upon information provided on the health history form. (Task)

- You focused your questions on the chief complaint of back pain. (Action)

- Asking what makes the back pain worse—or better—provided some insight into what might help the client. (Results)

This model does not have built-in opportunities for the student to provide a self-reflection. In some interpretations of this model, the A is used to identify "alternative" actions the student could have taken that would have achieved a different outcome. Taking that approach would invite self-reflection and an action plan.

Giving feedback to students in distance learning provides a dedicated opportunity for connection with students. Feedback sessions that are scheduled on a regular basis can be used to review general student progress. This can be helpful for students who may have difficulty keeping up or might lose motivation without face-to-face contact with the class. When specific feedback is provided to reflect upon or assess a learning activity it can help students feel acknowledged.

The entire arc of an educational program for exercise science or personal training is a transformative experience. As students acquire new knowledge, apply what they have learned, and keep an eye on a graduation date, they many not recognize transformation that occurs along the way. Using a combination of assessments, feedback, and opportunities for self-reflection can help students appreciate how they have grown and what they have learned.

Moving Beyond Lecturing

Distance learning is maturing and evolving. Instructors and students are recognizing that some approaches may be more effective than others to meet different learning objectives. What works for a face-to-face class does not always translate into the online environment. Live online lectures might meet contact hour requirements, but offer few opportunities for interaction and active engagement.

To simulate the live online lecture experience try sitting in front of a computer or television and watching a lengthy documentary on an unfamiliar topic. Stay within sight of the screen at all times and try to look attentive. Focus on the content. At the end reflect on how much information is retained. Probably not enough to pass a test. A live online lecture offers students a similar experience. It might be a convenient way to reach a large group of students, but is likely not effective to meet learning objectives.

Planning, practice, and patience are important for lecture-based instructors to move into active learning. Instructional strategies need to be suited to the course material, instructor, and level of students. The instructor should feel comfortable facilitating the format. Students should be willing—and able—to participate. Finding instructional strategies that are a good fit requires experimentation.

Finding Inspiration

In recent years there has been substantial innovation in distance teaching and learning. A wide range of courses provide examples of different structures and methods. Finding samples and examples can provide inspiration and ideas for engaging instruction. A little time spent doing some research can be very rewarding.

Certifications exist for everything, including distance learning, team-based learning, and problem-based learning. Getting trained or certified can be helpful to build a toolkit. But in some cases, the process is long and time consuming. Unless an institution requires training or certification to implement an instructional strategy, it may not be a worth the investment of time and money.

Conferring with colleagues can provide inspiration. Find out what they are doing in their courses. Ask what works well and where there are challenges. Probe a little deeper to inquire what they would like to do differently—and whether there are barriers to making changes. Ask for a tour of their virtual classroom. Look for the overall learning arc to see how the various components fit together.

Reaching out to educators in other disciplines can be helpful. Although the instructional material will be different, they may provide insight into using digital assets from publishers or integrating apps. Instructors that have worked with librarians to create a course reserve for library materials can share insights into the process.

Other schools and programs can be sources of inspiration. Course catalogues provide descriptions. Some instructors have public webpages with information on their courses and teaching strategies. Entering a course name followed by "syllabus" in an internet browser can sometimes turn up a few samples. It is important to remember that digitally accessed information—even when it is easy to obtain—may be subject to copyright. Open educational resources can be tapped for ideas.

Another opportunity to get inspiration is to be a student. Sign up to take a distance learning course. Enroll in a massive open online course (MOOC.) The non-credit options are generally offered at no cost. Courses in this group are most often asynchronous. The enrollment can be enormous with students from around the world. The instructional strategies used might not offer inspiration for ways to engage students. Something MOOCs do well is course organization so students can easily follow along.

Signing up for a non-academic course is another possibility. Courses that promote a hobby or skill (e.g. drawing, playing a musical instrument, or using Photoshop) balance demonstration with instruction. The presenters work hard to make the topics interesting in order to draw a following and boost their enrollment. The instructional approaches they use might inspire new active learning strategies. Navigating the virtual classrooms used in different eLearning platforms can build confidence.

Course Development

There is a somewhat pervasive myth that it takes a year to develop an online course. On average there are 2,087 work hours per calendar year. That seems an excessive amount of time to create a course with 135 total instructional hours! Many different factors contribute to the amount of time and effort needed for course development and instructional design. Teaching contracts often do not permit a lot of lead time before a course starts. Course assignments can change at the last minute. Instructors need to consider the timeline, costs, and effort in relation to other responsibilities. If the goal is to migrate a course to online or hybrid, starting on a small scale to replace lecture-based teaching with more engaging instructional strategies can make it less overwhelming.

Before instructors make major revisions to a course—or attempt to develop a new course—review by an administrative or institutional committee may be required. An accreditation agency may have guidelines specific for distance learning. Instructors should take time to become familiar with all requirements before developing a course or making major changes.

Choosing Instructional Strategies

Context and purpose are important for adult learners. Students who are used to sitting in lectures and taking tests may be resistant to other instructional approaches that require active participation. Students who thrive on interaction may welcome the opportunity to participate in active learning instead of sitting in a lecture. When a face-to-face class unexpectedly moves online (due to inclement weather or a global pandemic) instructors may need to make an effort to draw students into the distance learning classroom. Instructional design specifically for distance learning can take a creative approach to optimize engagement.

Designing a course using a formula for each session can help students navigate the class. This could be any combination of learning activities that meet course objectives. Consistently using a flipped classroom lets students know they need to arrive to live class meetings prepared. Pairing a book chapter with a quiz, using prerecorded lectures and a team debate, or incorporating a kinesthetic activity in every class requires engagement. When the formula is familiar it can maximize instructional time because students will know where to go and what to do.

For structured sessions that facilitate engagement, start by selecting an instructional strategy that feels comfortable. Sketch out a lesson plan. Include the learning objective(s) or learning outcome(s) for the session, identify materials that will be used, and the amount of time available. Next draw the learning arc to illustrate how the activity will build and where it should lead. Then identify informal assessments and formative assessment to give feedback to students and get feedback from them.

To design time for small groups, using short periods of time interspersed with whole class interaction can be beneficial. This helps maintain a connection and keeps students on task. The whole class interactions also help to ensure that all students have a similar learning opportunity through access to the same information. This is especially important when composition of small groups is uneven.

Pilot Testing

When instructors are ready to implement a new instructional strategy, a good rule of thumb is to try it three times. The first time will serve as an introduction to what the instructional strategy looks like and how it can be executed. The second time is a pilot test of the activity. The third session offers the opportunity for students and instructor to do it to actually experience the activity and achieve learning goals. Generally it takes a few weeks for a new course to settle in as students and instructors get to know their way around. Interspersing non-lecture activities in between lecture-based sessions gives time to help everyone get acclimated to requirements to be more involved during class time.

Course Evaluation

Institutions and programs use different methods and approaches to evaluate courses and instructors. A holistic evaluation is a combination of student evaluations, assessments of student performance, self-assessment by the instructor, and observation of teaching. Information provided in the different aspects of assessment help instructors and administration identify opportunities to refine content and instructional strategies.

Conducting observations of teaching in an online course is important so instructors receive feedback on their teaching. In face-to-face classes, when an observer attends for the purposes of evaluating the instructor, the observer is typically introduced. The reason for his/her attendance in the class is explained, and the observer maintains a discreet position for the duration of the class session. This is slightly more difficult to execute in distance learning because the observer must be temporarily invited into a course for the observation.

Technology help may be needed in order for a course to accommodate a guest for purposes of observing the instructor. Once that is achieved, the same approach can be taken for the observation as is customary in a face-to-face class. The observer's presence can be acknowledged and then he/she can maintain a discreet position in the background. If attending a synchronous course session, that might involve turning off the webcam so as not to be visibly distracting. When the learning activities include discussion forums, it would be useful for the observer to read through the entire forum just as they would listen to a live discussion in class. That would provide insight into how the instructor guides the tone of the conversation and uses discussion to teach. If the learning activities include small group work, it may not be feasible (or logical) for the observer to drop into groups alongside the instructor. Shadowing would require technical support. Once the observation is concluded, the observer should be removed from the course.

Evaluation of distance learning or hybrid courses should pay specific attention to the delivery (i.e. the LMS, instructional strategies, communication.) When students are given an option for a course offered online, face-to-face, or as a hybrid a comparative evaluation of the courses may be useful. If there are considerable differences in student evaluations or performance in the course that can indicate a need for more robust analysis of the delivery and instructional approaches.

Closing the Door

After a distance learning course has ended, the door to the virtual classroom should be closed. Students can take what they learned and apply it to subsequent courses or in professional practice. Instructors should follow institution, program, and accreditation guidelines to maintain grade records for the necessary length of time. All other aspects of the distance learning course should be archived after grades are issued. The digital record of course activities should be maintained, but there generally is no need to leave the virtual classroom open. This is important to maintain privacy and confidentiality for the students.

Before the end of a course students should be reminded to download and save all instructional materials. Completed assignments and worksheets may be helpful for review later on. A copy of the syllabus might come in handy later on if a student ever wants to apply for transfer credit for a course.

If instructors created the course materials, they should already have digital copies of tests, assignments, and discussion questions. But a copy of the final gradebook should be stored in a digitally secure file. If a student appeals a grade or needs to resolve an incomplete the instructor will be able to easily access information. It can also be helpful for instructors to review if they are called upon to write recommendation letters for students. The most important thing to remember for files that contain student information is that they must be stored securely.

For a CMS that is set up like a membership-based platform (e.g. Teachable, Thinkific) the default in the course design is to allow lifetime access. That means a course is open in perpetuity and can be accessed at any time by all who enrolled. If discussions or student-to-student interactions are used it can be confusing if it creates the perception that a student is interacting with someone who is no longer involved in the course. An ethical way to deal with this is to omit student-to-student interaction for staggered enrollment or asynchronous courses and instead use self-paced learning. Across higher education, it is not unusual to allow students extra time to complete a self-paced course. A specific time limit is generally used and access to a course is configured so it is limited to a defined period of time. Instruction can still include active learning to optimize student engagement. Upon completion, students should exit the course.

Conclusions

The term distance learning applies to any instruction that does not have instructors and students in the same place and space at the same time. Distance learning is not synonymous with online learning. Distance learning is a broader concept in that it recognizes the whole array of methods and materials used to connect, teach, and learn including—and beyond—the LMS.

The ability for instructors and students to interact with each other in different ways creates a range of possibilities for instructional design. Some activities are the same as those used in face-to-face courses (e.g. group projects, quizzes.) Others are unique to the distance learning environment (e.g. discussion forums, video essays.) As instructors gain experience in distance learning they will recognize that instructional activities and methods of assessment that work well in a face-to-face class do not necessarily work well online—and vice versa.

Redesigning a course can seem daunting. This is especially true for a course that has temporarily moved online. Yet that should not stop instructors from seeking out the best teaching strategies. A temporary adjustment in design or delivery might provide some inspiration for some innovation even after the course returns to in-person delivery.

Instructors who are seeking to move beyond lectures might want to start out small. This can be as simple as choosing a specific unit, module, or session and selecting an active learning strategy and writing a lesson plan. Rehearse the activity, give the students a guideline and then try it out. Immediately afterward assess and evaluate in relation to learning outcomes and the extent to which everyone felt more engaged with each other. Compare that to a routine lecture. It may take some experimentation to identify which instructional strategies work best for participants and course content.

Index

102, 145, 151, 152, 166, 167
SCORM, 27
Self-assessment, 179
Self-directed, 11, 22, 23, 24, 53, 64, 85, 86, 107, 141
Simulation, 36, 72, 120, 121, 122, 123, 124, 126
Software, 4, 19, 29, 45, 61, 143, 150, 163
Summative assessment, 83, 175, 176, 180
Supplemental resource, 39, 40, 116, 180
Synchronous, 9, 10, 12, 58, 64, 75, 90, 94, 103, 121, 144, 145,

152, 158, 163, 166, 168, 205
Technology, 3, 8, 10, 14, 17, 19, 28, 29, 50, 142, 144, 150, 152, 163, 164
Textbook, 28, 43, 44, 78, 81, 83, 85, 86, 95, 97, 98, 119
Time management, 4, 11, 153, 168
Vocational, 15, 16, 17, 21
Webcam, 1, 10, 29, 30, 42, 50, 59, 129, 132, 135, 136, 144, 150, 151, 159, 171, 172, 205
Workload, 4, 53, 56, 57, 58, 172

About the Author

Virginia S. Cowen, PhD is a researcher, writer, and educator with over 20 years' experience in health, fitness and wellness. She has been a member of the faculty at Rutgers University, the University of Medicine and Dentistry of New Jersey, and Queensborough Community College. Dr. Cowen earned her PhD in curriculum and instruction with a concentration in exercise and wellness from Arizona State University. She is a Google Certified Educator Level 1 and Level 2. She holds certifications as a strength and conditioning specialist (NSCA), personal trainer (ACE), Pilates teacher, and yoga teacher, and is also a licensed and board certified massage therapist. Dr. Cowen is passionate about education innovation.

Other Books by Virginia S. Cowen, PhD

Hands Off! 70 Active Learning Strategies for Exercise Science and Personal Training —Pennate Press

101 Cases for Study in Exercise Science and Personal Training —Pennate Press

Hands Off! 70 Active Learning Strategies for Massage and Bodywork Education —Pennate Press

Beyond Lectures: Engaging Distance Learning in Massage and Bodywork Education —Pennate Press

101 Cases for Study in Massage and Bodywork Education —Pennate Press

Hands Off! 70 Active Learning Strategies for Pilates Teacher Training —Pennate Press

Beyond Lectures: Engaging Distance Learning in Pilates Teacher Training —Pennate Press

101 Cases for Study in Pilates Teacher Training —Pennate Press

Hands Off! 70 Active Learning Strategies for Yoga Teacher Training —Pennate Press

101 Cases for Study in Yoga Teacher Training —Pennate Press

Pathophysiology for Massage Therapists: A Functional Approach —F.A. Davis

Therapeutic Massage and Bodywork for Autism Spectrum Disorders: A Guide for Parents and Caregivers—Singing Dragon Books

www.ingramcontent.com/pod-product-compliance
Lightning Source LLC
Chambersburg PA
CBHW070417270326
41926CB00014B/2832